Plagued

Plagued

PANDEMICS *from the*
BLACK DEATH *to* COVID-19
and BEYOND

John Froude, MD

BenBella Books, Inc.
Dallas, TX

BenBella

BenBella Books, Inc.
10440 N. Central Expressway
Suite 800
Dallas, TX 75231
benbellabooks.com
Send feedback to feedback@benbellabooks.com

BenBella is a federally registered trademark.

Printed in the United States of America
10 9 8 7 6 5 4 3 2 1

Library of Congress Cataloging-in-Publication Data is available upon request.
ISBN 9781950665754 (print)
ISBN 9781953295361 (ebook)

Image on page 90: Septemberlegs/Alamy Stock Photo.
Image on page 196 used with permission by Sarah Oquendo.
All other photography from the public domain.

Editing by Sheila Curry Oakes
Copyediting by Michael Fedison
Proofreading by Lisa Story and Cape Cod Compositors, Inc.
Indexing by Amy Murphy
Text composition by Yara Abuata
Cover design by Sarah Avinger
Printed by Lake Book Manufacturing

Special discounts for bulk sales are available.
Please contact bulkorders@benbellabooks.com.

To my children:
Abigail, Susannah, Jack, and Luke

And, of course, to the Fever Demon, Djvarasura

CONTENTS

"All the infections that the sun sucks up
From bogs, fens, flats
On Prosper fall and make him
By inch–meal a disease!"

~Caliban, **The Tempest,** *Act II, Scene 2*

INTRODUCTION

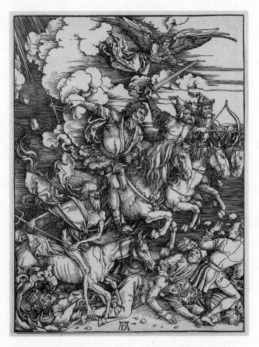

The Four Horsemen of the Apocalypse
by Albrecht Dürer (1471–1528).

Albrecht Dürer's masterwork *The Four Horsemen of the Apocalypse* offers a medieval view of life in his interpretation of the quartet from the book of Revelation. Death dominates the foreground. The horseman to his right represents Famine. Pestilence is shooting his arrows, a common metaphor throughout European-centered history for infection, notably bubonic plague, and War holds his sword ready. Famine, Pestilence, War, and Death. In the bottom left-hand corner, a mitred cleric is being swallowed headfirst by an apocalyptic beast, while ordinary men and women are trampled before the stampede. Above them all flies an angel with a beneficent gaze, the one glimmer of hope, but this creature of divinity is far away and up in the air. Might the angel represent reason? The advent of the enlightenment perhaps? Louis Pasteur?

Probably not.

These three great generals, Plague, Famine, and War, act in the service of Death. War and Plague are close comrades. They stalk the world today and have done so throughout history. Napoleon's army in Moscow was slaughtered by typhus. During the Napoleonic wars, in the British army, eight times more people died from disease than from battle wounds. Two-thirds of those who died in the American Civil War died of an infection, with dysentery, measles, and typhus the preeminent causes. During the Irish famine, people also suffered from smallpox, dysentery, and a typhus-like illness. Typhus slaughtered soldiers and civilians alike during the First and Second World Wars. More American soldiers died of influenza in the First World War than in battle. The contemporary war in Yemen has led to the largest cholera epidemic ever reported. Those affected by war include an estimated forty million refugees in the world today who are subject to infections caused by mass movement, poor sanitation, unclean drinking water, starvation, and the breakdown of structured society. They are afflicted by cholera, dysentery, malaria, pneumonia, measles, relapsing fever, tuberculosis, and AIDS.

When war comes along, you may take plagues for granted, but Pestilence stalks in peacetime, too. Though metaphors of war and battle are often invoked when speaking of plagues, they have been much more destructive than war. Plagues have killed hundreds of millions of us. They have been with us since the beginning, and they are with us still.

The word *plague* comes from the Greek word *plaga*, meaning "strike," as in strike a blow. It was borrowed by the Romans; *plaga* now signifying a little more: affliction with slaughter and destruction. It was first used to mean an outbreak of disease by the physician Galen in 210 CE. Its first English use was in the 14th century to describe the Black Death. *Plague* remained synonymous with the Black Death until the early 17th century when, with the advent of the King James Bible, the word began to be used more generally to mean any widespread life-threatening calamity—

including lethal fever-producing diseases. Now it is also synonymous with the word *pandemic*, an infectious disease outbreak spread over many countries or the world.

THE PONIES OF THE APOCALYPSE

The invisible creatures that cause plagues—viruses, bacteria, and protists using us as energy sources to replicate—couldn't strike their blows alone. They require a supporting force, and that force is us.

Plagues don't travel—they ride. They ride with *Homo sapiens*, on birds, in bats, and with many land animals. It is all too easy to find examples of traveling armies spreading disease, of colonizers bringing pandemic destruction with them, of trade along all the Silk Roads of the planet, ships crewed by men closely packed together, or trains instigating outbreaks by carrying people from distant places to the metropolis, and ships spreading infection from seaport to seaport. Smallpox spread around the world in about two hundred years. It took syphilis fifty. Spanish flu started in one location and was found across the globe within a year.

About 4.54 billion people flew on commercial airlines in 2019, making flight a potent disseminator of plagues. SARS-CoV-2 spread to almost every country in the world from one place—Wuhan, China—in four months. That is not a property of the virus, it is an attribute of the airplane.

In our global world there isn't a bacterium or a virus more than twelve hours away from any other spot on Earth. Thus, airplane travel is one in a stable of apocalyptic ponies that may participate in any illness-fueled stampede, whether riding alone or alongside the horses of War or Famine. How they work depends on time and place, but each of these apocalyptic ponies has acted and will act again in the service of the plague master, Death:

- Movement of populations through travel, invasion, exploration, and trade—exposing new people to new pathogens
- Crowded living conditions, whether for armies or civilians
- Unsanitary conditions and inadequate disposal of human waste

- Contaminated drinking water
- Poor control of mosquitos and other pests (fleas, rodents)
- Ignorance, delusion (e.g., AIDS denialism), or plain stupidity (i.e., not using available control methods)
- Superstitions or religious beliefs that resist science
- Ethnocentricity, scapegoating
- Unsterilized needles, unprotected sex, sexual tourism
- Political incompetence or corruption
- Natural disasters
- Climate change
- Proximity to animals, particularly primates

Like the first pony on the list, travel, the last also deserves particular attention. Of the ninety known bacteria and 220 viruses so far shown to cause infections in humans, three-quarters are "zoonoses"—diseases we share, acquire, or have acquired from non-human animals. The word was coined by the great 19th-century German pathologist Rudolf Virchow who went on to say, "Between animal and human medicine, there is no dividing line, nor should there be."

There is an animal presence in Dürer's woodcut. Horses can transmit infections to man, including rabies, encephalitis caused by at least three viruses, plus a fourth called equine encephalitis that killed two hundred thousand horses and several thousand humans in Mexico and Texas in 1971. In the single year of 1995 in Colombia, one hundred thousand people suffered from these infections. Other infections that can pass to humans from horses include: influenza virus, salmonella, glanders, melioidosis, anthrax, brucellosis, babesiosis, leptospirosis, horse measles, and hydatid disease. These illnesses are rare in our developed world, but they would have been troublesome and relevant on the Pontic-Caspian steppe seven thousand years ago where horses were first domesticated. Hendra virus is named after a suburb of Brisbane, Australia, where, in 1994, it caused an acute febrile respiratory illness that infected at least twenty-one horses, fourteen of which had to be put down, and two humans, one of whom died.

There are 4,000 living species of mammal. The single largest group are rodents, with 1,500 species. The second most frequent are Chiroptera, also known as bats, with 1,000 species. Both these groups are natural reservoirs for pathogens, and sixty-one viruses have been identified in bats and sixty-eight in rodents to date. Bats may be chronically infected but show no sign of disease. From time to time, they shed virus. Paleovirology suggests that infections now seen only in humans such as measles, smallpox, and mumps had their origins in bats. They are the first home of rabies, Ebola, coronaviruses, and many others.

Homo sapiens is also an enabler of plagues in animals, which is known as *reverse* zoonoses. Cattle acquired tuberculosis from man. Influenza from a human recently killed six bonobos in a Congo wildlife sanctuary. Swine, birds, and humans cross-infect with influenza. Plagues in non-human animals follow a similar pattern to plagues in *H sapiens* and are influenced by identical environmental variables. If three-quarters of our infections are zoonoses, the remaining 25 percent come from contaminated drinking water polluted with human or animal detritus.

We are somewhat aware that we are animals. Many of us pretend we aren't. At least we try not to draw attention to it. Our animal nature is shrouded in euphemism. This modesty or boastfulness must be abandoned when thinking about human infections. Our diseases and our control of them, our living or dying from infection, depends on acknowledging ourselves as just one more animal species. Fully 98 percent of our DNA is shared with the chimpanzee, the sooty mangabey, and the bonobo—our closest animal relatives. That 2 percent difference between us and the chimp has led to some pretty astounding artifacts, it must be said: St Peter's in Rome, the Boeing 747, penicillin, your laptop, books, the bicycle, and a bomb that can destroy an entire city. A plague is not fully described until the animals involved in its origin, those that get infected, those that act as reservoirs, and those that transmit infection are also identified. When a plague begins, look for the animals and remember your own animal nature.

———————

This book describes eleven infectious plagues that have scourged mankind and the one through which we are living, COVID-19. Among the twelve is an account of the Spanish flu that began just over a century ago, which has been called the Mother of All Pandemics. Over this short one hundred years, our knowledge of viruses, bacteria, protists, epidemiology, immunity, evolution, genetics, and medicine has grown at a phenomenal rate. But we also know only too well that a plague is much more than a clinical description in a textbook of infectious diseases. A plague brings sociological, financial, domestic, and political consequences.

It is the aim of *Plagued* to shed light on what plagues us: What is our exact biological relationship with microbes? Why do we have plagues? How are they and must they be reevaluated as we acquire new knowledge? Finally, while we now understand plagues better than ever, we continue to contribute to their virulence and persistence through the apocalyptic horsemen and their large stable of ponies: In the global village that the world has become, how will we prevent, treat, and control the plagues of the future?

For more plagues will come.

CHAPTER I

....

VIRGIN SOIL: PANDEMICS AND IMMUNITY

T he first people to cross the Bering Land Bridge from Siberia to Alaska in 20,000 BCE would not have thought, nor could they have known, that they were the first humans to enter two continents amounting to a quarter of the world's land mass and teeming with edible life. Some crossed and then returned to Asia. Some lived on the Bridge for a few thousand years.

It would be thirteen thousand years before the first Europeans, Eric the Red and his fellow Norsemen, reached the continent. They sailed to Greenland in 985. Perhaps there were earlier travelers that we don't know of. We do know that by 1491, there were fifty million people living in the territory from Alaska to Tierra del Fuego as these places are known today.

Countless tribal identities and languages developed across the Americas. Half lived in what is now Mexico. Tenochtitlan, the capital of the Aztecs, was larger than Madrid or London in 1500, and represented an advanced civilization.

IMMUNOGLOBULIN G, THE ANTIBODY THAT CHANGED THE WORLD

The human immune system is a magic cloak that you don't know you have until it's torn. It is extremely complex, imperfect, and a constant evolutionary work in progress. It is marshaled by a network of highly specialized cells that identify microbes, eliminate them, and develop a molecular record to better deal with future exposure, should they return.

We cannot live without it. The clinical manifestations of the three or four hundred diseases caused by microbes are the result of interaction between immunity and pathogen.

Take the common boil. It is red, hot, tender, and swollen. The pus you squeeze out of it is the debris of an interaction between the staphylococcus pumping out toxins as it multiplies under your skin and the white blood cells that have evolved to engulf and destroy the bacteria—often dying in the process.

There are also microbes that used to cause disease but do not do so now as long as our immunity is intact. AIDS occurs when the immune system is severely damaged by the human immunodeficiency virus (HIV). AIDS patients get secondarily infected with common microbes found in the atmosphere like *Pneumocystis jerovicki* and *Mycobaterium avium intracellulare* that do not cause illness at all in immunocompetent people.

Your immune system defends against infection at three levels. Think of it as three walls around a castle. The outer wall is a barrier. This is skin, mucous membranes, the stomach's acid milieu, the little cilia on the bronchial mucosa of the airways that waft particulate matter upwards and out through coughing. As you will know from the experience of having a head cold, there can be outpourings of mucus in the nose to flush the invader away.

If the outer wall is broken by a cut in the skin, a needle in a vein, or the microbe cunningly attaching to the mucosa (as happens with the influenza virus, which uses the cell's own enzymes to enter it), then the first defenses are down.

In the bloodstream, bacteria double and redouble in the nutrient-rich environment. Viruses multiply in the cytoplasm or nucleus of a cell; different cells for different viruses. They use the cell's machinery to mass-produce themselves, then exit to infect other cells. Cells thus infected vary from virus to virus. SARS-CoV-2 will enter any cell with the ACE2 receptor on it. These are found mostly in the nose, mouth, and lungs but also in the heart, kidneys, liver, nervous tissue, and gastrointestinal tract.

The second level of immune defense counterattacks. *Cytokines*, messenger molecules, are released from many cells, particularly those called Helper T Cells found in the blood, lymph nodes, or the spleen. They activate a range of other specialized cells triggering inflammation and engulfing the intruder. Acute phase antibodies, immunoglobulin M (IgM), freshly synthesized in the blood's plasma cells, bind to the microbe, incapacitating it. There is a cascade of specific proteins, called the complement system, that flow around bacteria, making it easier for the white blood cells to engulf them. This cascade constructs little missiles called Membrane Attack Complexes (MACs) that puncture holes in the walls of bacteria, killing them.

This complexity of the immune response requires detailed study to describe thoroughly, and even then, our knowledge is incomplete. This is what is happening inside the body on a cellular level. On the outside, depending on the pathogen, you see fever, exhaustion, malaise, loss of appetite, aches in muscles, pain in joints, a rash, a runny nose, a headache, delirium, and diarrhea. The patient is incapacitated until death or survival. If you survive this inner molecular confrontation, you start to feel better yet easily tire. This is convalescence, the calm after the storm.

Immunity does not stop there. This is not simply a knockout ten-round fight between immune system and pathogen. The third level of resistance is *adaptive immunity*. Specific immunoglobulin G (IgG) is an antibody made, like IgM, in cellular factories called plasma cells. Having been infected and having survived, the IgG your body makes will protect you against reinfection. If you have survived smallpox, measles, or many other infectious diseases, you can never have them a second time. Your specific IgG neutralizes these pathogens. You are immune. The way immunoglobin G functions is the basis for vaccination, which stimulates the adaptive immune system without infection, leaving behind immunity.

IgG represents 75 percent of antibodies. With its two binding sites, it wraps up viruses, bacteria, and the few protozoa and fungi that can cause disease in humans. It neutralizes toxins.

However, IgG doesn't work for every infection. As immunity evolves, so does the microbe in a never-ending arms race. Influenza virus rotates its outer proteins, so each variant is perceived by the immune system as a new infection. Some infections induce partial immunity. If you survive malaria, for example, your second infection will be milder.

The result of this biochemical interaction in your body spells the difference between life and death.

Life in Europe in 1492 was precarious. Famine in the countryside led the poor to the cities where the decomposing offal of butchered animals lay in the streets, ditches were used as public latrines, and overcrowding and poverty predominated. The continent was rife with the Horsemen and their ponies.

In the overcrowded houses where many slept in one bed, children, like children everywhere, were born with protective IgG that had crossed the placenta from their mothers. This protects for the first year of life, but then it wears off so that they are highly susceptible to measles, smallpox, chicken pox, whooping cough, mumps, influenza, tuberculosis, and ague (malaria). Half of all children born in those days died before the age of ten. Every twenty years or so, bubonic plague, typhus, and dysentery, with an overall 10 to 30 percent mortality, broke out in the expanding cities. In the 1500s, if you survived to a ripe old age of fifty, your immunity would wane. Fifty was a reasonable life expectancy among the rich and well fed, but it was much lower for everyone else. Infection was the cause of nearly all deaths, but if you survived, you would develop immunity or partial immunity mediated by IgG.

And, as a survivor, you might yearn to explore new worlds and to leave your disease-ridden and poverty-stricken old world behind.

COLUMBUS'S SECOND VOYAGE

Columbus left Cadiz for his second voyage to the New World on September 24, 1493. On this occasion, he had seventeen galleons and caravels and twelve hundred men, including half a dozen priests. As before, he was looking for India, silver, and gold. He also had another mission—to colonize Hispaniola and dominate its inhabitants known as the Taino.

The islands that he had "discovered" were ripe for cultivation, and the "natives" could do the work. He also wanted to restore contact with the forty crewmen left behind from his first voyage following the shipwreck of the *Santa Maria*.

He stopped at the Canary Islands for a month and took horses, sheep, cattle, and eight sows on board. These were the first pigs to be taken to the "Indies." His fleet crossed the Atlantic in the speedy time of three weeks, and he began looking for a place to put his plantation while he explored these islands of paradise. On December 7, 1493, he established a settlement on the north coast of Hispaniola. He called it La Isabela. As the fleet unloaded, he learned that the crew of the *Santa Maria* were all dead, killed, it was said, by the Taino.

As the pigs were driven off the boat, people began to fall ill. They sickened with exhaustion and malaise followed by high fevers of abrupt onset. Later, there were runny noses and chest pain. Columbus himself caught the disease and was unwell for a month. Over the next two weeks, three hundred Spaniards died. As unexpected as this loss of life was, it was nothing compared to the mortality of the Taino who lost two-thirds of their number. The disease spread through Hispaniola and onto the nearby islands named Cuba and Puerto Rico by the Spaniards.

In 1535, Gonzalo Fernández de Oviedo wrote the *General History of the Indies*. He describes the epidemic:

Half the Spanish were dead and so many Indians died that they could not be counted. And this happened in a way that could not be understood or any remedy put to it . . . and in this way all through the land the Indians lay dead everywhere. The stench was very great and pestiferous.

Of the twelve hundred men who had set out from Cadiz in 1494, only three hundred were still alive in 1502. We don't know the size of the Taino population. A reasonable estimate of a million people has been made. *More fell daily everywhere like cattle in a sicken herd, hard to imagine how many had been killed. They die very easily from disease,* wrote Pietro Martyr Anglerius in 1500. So many died, they could not be counted. Many were killed by soldiers or died of starvation, but most died from infection.

Scholars disagree as to the cause of the illness, and in the absence of objective evidence, we will never know. Influenza and typhus are the main suspects, and of the two, suspicion falls on influenza because of the imported swine.

By the time smallpox came to Hispaniola, twenty-six years later, the Taino population was eight thousand, and by 1535, they were extinct.

The swine ran the hills in large herds.

PAWTUXET

Fast-forward to 1619. As Tisquantum watched from the deck of Master Dermer's open pinnacle, his emotions were profound. Having sailed from Newfoundland, they now approached the natural harbor of Pawtuxet, soon to be named Plymouth, on the coast of Dawnland, soon to be called New England. Four years earlier, he had been kidnapped for the second time on this shore, taken to Spain, and sold into slavery. He was fortunate to be freed by a group of Franciscan friars. They helped him sail to London where he had but one thought in his mind—to get home.

He was taken under the wing of Captain Slaney in the London Docks, treasurer of the Newfoundland Company and a shipbuilder. Slaney liked Tisquantum because he had learned English. He could see that "Squanto" would be useful as an interpreter in the settlements in Newfoundland.

Now, in May, Tisquantum was returning to Pawtuxet. He had heard rumors. There was talk of a plague among the "savages." It turned out to be more than talk. As they sailed along the coast, they stopped at previously busy ports known to him from earlier years. Each town was now depopulated with only a few broken survivors. They found caches of abandoned crops, tools, and other supplies. The fields were untended. A plague had wiped out the Massachussets, Penacook, Nauset, Permaquid, and Abenaki tribes and Tisquantum's own tribe, the Wampanoag.

For the preceding three years, a pestilence had been raging among the indigenous peoples. What was terrible and unexplainable to them was that the French, the Dutch, and the English with whom they mingled and traded were not affected. Why was it not killing these white people from the Eastern Ocean? This latest plague was the worst. It extended along a two-hundred-mile coastline and at least fifteen miles inland. Thomas Morton, a witness to the devastation, writes,

> *For in a place where many inhabited, there hath been but one left a live, to tell what became of the rest, the living beings (as it seems) not able to bury the dead, they were left for the Crowes, Kites and vermin to prey upon . . . it seemed to me a new found Golgotha.*

When Tisquantum landed in Pawtuxet, the town was deserted. He ran from familiar place to familiar place searching for a sign of life, and at the top of the lookout hill he came across a large number of skeletons, without order. They had not been buried as was the custom.

This was his homecoming.

Master Dermer persuaded him to go into the interior. He would need Tisquantum's services as an interpreter. They passed some ancient settlements, previously populous, now deserted. After three days' journey, they found the inhabited village of Namaskut.

Since the slaving raid that had abducted Tisquantum, a powerful hatred had arisen between the indigenous Americans and the Europeans. So much so that when a French fishing ship ran aground on Cape Cod three years previously, most of the few survivors were killed. Two were enslaved and one died shortly after, but not before invoking a divine curse upon his captors.

"Puisse Dieu vous frappez morts"—May God strike you dead.

In the village of Namaskut, Dermer recorded, *They would have killed me, except Squanto entreated hard for my life.* Relationships improved slowly as Dermer "redeemed," or bought back, the enslaved Frenchman.

Here, Tisquantum learned the full extent of the epidemic. In Dermer's later account, *Thousands of them died, they not being able to burie one another, their sculs and bones were found in many places lying still above ground a sad spectacle to behold. Not one in twenty survived.* Such survivors as there were, were sick and wasted with sores. The illness started with severe headache, then fever, then "yellowness" all over the body, bleeding from the nose, collapse, and death. Through the eye of history, the death toll of this epidemic on the Eastern Seaboard of North America, 1616–1619, is estimated at sixty thousand.

Various theories for the causes of the plague arose: A comet had been seen. There was an earthquake somewhere that had changed the air. It had come from Egypt. The usual suspects were cited, but the Pilgrims had no doubts—it was the Hand of God. They saw their lives as parallel to the Israelite exodus from Egypt. As Daniel Denton wrote some years later,

The hand of God eminently seen. Making consumption upon some Indian nations, as if God had an intention speedily to plant an English settlement. It hath generally been observed that when the English come to settle, a divine hand makes way for them. The wonderful and unsearchable Providence of GOD in the whole affair of driving out the natives for their sins and detestable vices.

The Pilgrim fathers arrived in Cape Cod, Massachusetts, on November 11, 1620, and eventually settled in Pawtuxet, renaming it Plymouth and establishing their colony. They were not the first Europeans to the northeastern shore of North America by any means. For a hundred years or more, Portuguese, Breton, and Bristol fishermen; Basque whalers; French fur traders and English codders; Spanish adventurers and speculators of every stripe had plied these waters, bringing bacteria and viruses with them into a virgin soil.

Plymouth wasn't the first English settlement. That honor belongs to Jamestown, Virginia, not counting the failed colonies of Roanoke and Merrymount. The Plymouth colony endured. These Puritan separatists ultimately became firmly established in the cultural imagination of the United States of America and its annual Thanksgiving celebration.

When Tisquantum heard of the newest Europeans' arrival at Plymouth, he went to meet them, no doubt astonishing them with his English. He showed them how best to use the local resources to plant corn and fish. He attended that first Thanksgiving, listening as they sang the "Old Hundredth." Subsequent portrayals of the feast show at least one "Native American" with two feathers in his hair. That is how Squanto is known to every American schoolchild.

Although the colony survived, life was not easy for the colonists. From November 1620 to March 1621, fully 49 of the 102 people who left Plymouth, England, died from a mixture of scurvy, pneumonia, and tuberculosis. Half of the thirty crewmembers of the *Mayflower* also died in less than six months.

Tisquantum settled with the Pilgrims, having no other family. Two years later, he sickened and, in a few days, died from what was ironically called "Indian Fever." The source of his illness was a bacteria or a virus carried by the Europeans in their blood and breath to this virgin population. Between the slaughter of the Taino on Hispaniola in 1495 to the death of Tisquantum in Pawtuxet-Plymouth in 1629, repeated epidemics led to catastrophic loss of life among the indigenous peoples. Most historians accept that 90 percent of the fifty million died. After the Taino, the Aztecs, the Incas, the Mayans, and peoples as far north as Florida and southern Georgia perished from infection brought by the Spanish and the Portuguese. To the north, it was the British who brought the microbes.

Europeans, their blood alive with specific IgG, brought disease after disease with them to which they were immune or were less sickened when infected. The only explanation that could be found for these mystifying events was that it was God's will that the Europeans should have the land. But was it God's will that the indigenous labor force was to disappear? In 1518, Emperor Charles V, grandson of Ferdinand and Isabella, authorized the transport of African slaves to Santo Domingo.

This is not to say that the mortality was entirely due to infection. In David E. Stannard's *American Holocaust*, he details the slaughter, the massacres, the dismemberment, and enslavement of the indigenous peoples at the hands of the Spanish, Portuguese, and British colonizers that continued over the next three hundred years with acts of genocide that could not have been pursued with such enthusiasm had not disease already weakened the population. The slaughter of these peoples remains the greatest loss of life due to war, disease, and genocide recorded in human history.

The decimation of native-born populations was not unique to the Americas. Everywhere the European colonizers went, the indigenous people died in huge numbers. It appeared that none could survive the onslaught of the Europeans and their microbes—the Maoris of New Zealand, the Aborigines of Australia, the Inuit of Canada, and the inhabitants of India.

Virgin soil epidemics probably occurred in Europe first. *Who We Are and How We Got Here* by Harvard professor David Reich has analyzed ancient DNA from many skeletal remains across the continent. He uncovers an interesting truth. Five thousand years ago, in relatively recent times, Europe was populated first by farmers who were sufficiently technically advanced to build Stonehenge. They flourished. Yet hardly any of their genes are to be found in modern-day Europeans. They are represented to the same extent that Taino genes are represented in the inhabitants of the Caribbean, which is not extensively. There are no pure-blood indigenous people remaining.

These first farmers in Europe were replaced by the Yamnaya, steppe people who had mastered the horse and the wheel five thousand years ago. By exploiting these discoveries, which were as momentous then as the computer in our lifetime, they were able to expand utilization of the land. Seventy percent of all European genes come from them; over 80 percent of people in Ireland and Wales have the Yamnaya genetic marker. The Yamnaya came from what are now called Armenia and Iran—their genes present in equal proportion. They brought the Indo-European languages with them, were a male-centered culture, and carried huge hammer axes. They built burial mounds called kurgans in which some of their leaders were buried with horses and carriages.

The first farmers who lived on the land before the Yamnaya came knew how to fight, just like the Taino, the Aztecs, and the Mayans. They had an advanced society. Yet they disappeared without a trace, likely due to plague. The bubonic plague was endemic in Europe at that time, so the Yamnaya won with the plague to which they were relatively immune. Just like the conquistadores in the Americas.

Tribe X invades Tribe Y and defeats them easily because Tribe X is immune to the plague they bring with them. Neither Tribe X nor Tribe Y has any idea why these events are occurring and seeks to explain the discrepancy in bias-reinforcing theology.

The reverse may also happen. Tribe Y can be immune and the invading Tribe X vulnerable. This was the effect of malaria on the Europeans as they tried to colonize West Africa. Another example is the French invasion of Haiti ordered by Napoleon in 1802. He sent twenty thousand men to quash the latest slave uprising. The French had far superior forces, yet only three thousand were to survive and return to France. Most died from yellow fever and, to a lesser extent, malaria, infections in Haiti that were brought on slave ships and to which the inhabitants were immune or relatively immune. Twice as many French soldiers died in Haiti as died at the Battle of Waterloo. In direct consequence, Napoleon abandoned his ideas of expanding the empire into the Americas and sold the Louisiana Territory to the United States, doubling the size of that country with a pen stroke.

The slaughter that disease brought to the indigenous Americans is unparalleled in history. Their most hideous enemies were not the European invaders themselves, as bad as they were, but the invisible killers they brought with them.

Chapter 2

....

MASTERS OF THE PLANET: BACTERIA

W e are here because bacteria allow us to be. Bacteria appeared on the planet 3.8 billion years ago. All plant and animal life has evolved from them. We are their descendants. For 2.5 billion years, together with *archaea*, they were the only forms of life on Earth. Archaea are another group of single-celled organisms that differ in structure from bacteria and have not, so far, been shown to cause disease in humans.

Bacteria purify water, make the soil productive by metabolizing essential chemicals from environmental nitrogen, and contribute 150 billion kilograms/year of oxygen to the atmosphere, without which we could not breathe. If all humans on Earth died, life would continue, scarcely noticing. If all the bacteria on Earth died, all other life would come to an end within a few years.

In 2014, Micropia, a museum in Amsterdam, was opened to celebrate the *beneficial* side of bacteria. It is only a few kilometers away from the location where Antonie van Leeuwenhoek became the first person to see bacteria in 1668 through his invention, the light microscope. In the 350 years since van Leeuwenhoek first saw bacteria through the microscope he had invented, information as to the nature of these animalcules accrued slowly at first. It was 150 years before Louis Pasteur showed that they caused disease in humans and another 70 before his ideas were universally accepted.

In the 21st century, microbiologists have uncovered information about bacteria at an exponential rate. Yet they still have many secrets to yield. This is not a trivial pursuit. It was from bacteria and fungi that antibiotics were developed. *Deinococcus radiodurans* can survive ten thousand times the radiation dose that is lethal to humans, and *Ideonella sakaiensis* can break down and consume plastics in the ocean as a sole energy source.

We use bacteria to make alcohol, manufacture fertilizer, treat waste, break down oil spills, make cheese and yoghurt, and recover gold, palladium, copper, and other metals from ores by the process of "bio-leaching." They have no consciousness. As obvious as this is, their amazing adaptability gives the impression that they do. Bacteria have been replicating by binary fission every twenty minutes for three and a half billion years. We replicate once every 400 hours. In that time, an average bacterium has passed through 1,200 generations.

These ancient molecules have adapted to life in many environments. They can live in hot air vents deep beneath the ocean, in glacial Antarctic caves, in the geysers of Yellowstone Park, in your stomach where there is acid, and particularly in your colon. Ninety-nine percent of the organisms in our colon have yet to be classified, and the same applies to the myriad organisms in the oceans. Only a few cause diseases.

For someone like me, who has spent a lifetime combating infectious disease, the idea that bacteria can be friendly takes a bit of adjustment. Yet it has become abundantly clear that many of these bugs are *symbionts*. We need them. When we eat, they eat. When we travel, they come with. When we die, they consume us.

THE MICROBIOME

Bacteria join us at birth. Meconium, fetal feces, is sterile. Newborns acquire bacteria from the birth canal and later from food. By the age of three, we have acquired the full panoply of colonic, skin, and mucus membrane bacteria. We are each an ecosystem teeming and teaming with bacteria, viruses, protists, fungi, and archaea living in a close community collectively known as *the microbiome*. There are 39 billion individual organisms per person. Let me say that again: 39 thousand billion.

The National Institutes of Health has undertaken the Human Microbiome Project to characterize it by sequencing the DNA of its microbial contents. This began in 2004 and isn't finished yet. Astonishingly, 99 percent of all existing microbes whose DNA is detectable are uncultured and unnamed by science to date.

Microbes contribute 3.3 million microbial genes to an individual, with only 23,000 from the human genome. They contribute more genes responsible for human survival than humans themselves. These two genomes combine to make us a superorganism. Microbes differ so much from one individual to the next that they could be used for forensic purposes like fingerprints. They also differ depending on their location in and on the body. For example, the microbiome of the armpit is different from the microbiome of the forearm. Your armpit is likely to be more similar to someone else's armpit than to your forearm. The bacteria on our body contribute to body odor. Streptococci cause the cheesy smell of feet, pseudomonas smells like wine, and anaerobes provide the odor of a decomposing corpse.

The microbiome detoxifies carcinogens in the intestine. It breaks down other toxins and harmful chemicals. It helps us digest. It supplies vitamins, minerals, and trace elements that are missing from our diets. It crowds out dangerous microbes or kills them with locally secreted antibiotics. A key function of the microbiome is its dynamic relationship with immunity. In early life, it educates the developing immune system about the difference between friend and foe, self and other, and contributes to its maintenance through life.

The essential nature of bacteria is contrary to our idea of them as disease-causers, or *pathogens*: Most are either unknown, harmless, or helpful.

Those bacteria that cause disease have a survival strategy based on causing damage. Damage facilitates their spread and allows colonization in novel parts of the body. They have evolved toxins that destroy the integrity of the host cell membrane, that dysregulate immune cells, and produce the immune response of too much inflammation, which may cause further damage.

Two bacteria at the root of contemporary human pandemics are *Helicobacter pylori* and *Clostridium difficile*.

Helicobacter pylori

Our stomach produces acid to kill bacteria. *H pylori* lives there anyway. It infects approximately 75 percent of the human population. It has been with us for 58,000 years, an association that began in East Africa as established by DNA technology. Acquired mostly in childhood, by the fecal-oral route or by kissing, *H pylori* does not begin to reveal its effects until a person reaches forty years of age. It causes gastric ulcer and cancer of the stomach. It may also cause or contribute to the cause of skin diseases such as acne rosacea, urticaria (hives), lichen planus, and others. It has been implicated as a possible cause of a number of neurological, cardiac, and dermatological diseases, although these are hypotheses yet to be established or rejected.

Clostridium difficile

When Elizabeth O'Toole and Ivan Hall first discovered *Clostridium difficile* in 1935, they found it difficult to culture. Hence its name. In 2020, it is the most common hospital-acquired infection in the United States. When antibiotics are used to treat an infection, many bacteria in the colon are killed. This allows *C difficile*, which inhabits the microbiome and is resistant to many commonly used antibiotics, to flourish and dominate the microbes that remain. It secretes a powerful toxin that causes colitis characterized by diarrhea with blood and mucus that may be severe and potentially lethal. *C difficile* colitis is a very good reason to use antibiotics as sparingly as possible. It is particularly common in the elderly, perhaps as a consequence of waning immunity. Severe cases may be cured by fecal transplant—taking feces from a healthy donor and emulsifying them in a blender. It is then administered either as an enema or through a tube through the nose into the stomach. It repairs the imbalance of bacteria in the colon, and the treatment can be nothing short of lifesaving. This procedure is an example of a healthy microbiome being used to cure a sick one.

Militaristic metaphors appear apt when it comes to combating bacteria. We marshal forces to fight them and send battalions of therapies and vaccines to seek and destroy these invisible invaders. But their rate of replication permits rapid evolution, an example of which is bacteria's development of resistance to antibiotics over the last seventy years.

The significance of these *bugs* (medical jargon) cannot be overstated. They have led to the deaths of hundreds of millions of people since *H sapiens* appeared on Earth, and they continue to attack us. Human evolution of a highly complex immune system is a testament in itself to their significance. Some of the better-known bacteria are described in this book—*Yersinia pestis, Cholera suis, Mycobacterium tuberculosis*. Some have names recognized in everyday speech: salmonella, streptococci, staphylococci.

Bubonic plague, cholera, typhus, tuberculosis, and syphilis shall be discussed in the following chapters.

Of thirty thousand species of bacteria so far identified, fewer than a hundred cause disease. But when they do, what pandemics!

CHAPTER 3

....

DECIPHERING BLACK DEATH: BUBONIC PLAGUE

I t is 2014. In Colorado, not far from Boulder, a fifty-year-old man takes his sick pit bull terrier to a vet. The vet is puzzled by the animal's illness. "He's got bad pneumonia," he says. "I'm sorry, he has to be euthanized."

Two days later, the dog's owner falls ill with a fever and shortness of breath. When he reaches the hospital, he is immediately placed on a ventilator and taken to the Intensive Care Unit (ICU). A friend who had helped him with the pit bull also develops a high fever, as do two assistants from the vet's office. Routine bloodwork shows that all four have *Yersinia pestis* (*Y pestis*) growing in their blood streams.

Yersinia pestis is the bacteria that causes bubonic plague.

The bubonic plague, also known as the Black Death! The one plague that everyone has heard of. It killed fifty million people in Europe, half of the population, in the Dark Ages. It conjures up images of red crosses painted on the doors of the afflicted, piles of skulls, and cries of "Bring out your dead." The plague ravaged Europe in the 14th century, so how do four Americans and a dog living in our contemporary, hygienic world get infected with this medieval scourge?

The bacteria discovered in the blood of these unlucky people from Colorado have a family tree stretching back for twenty thousand years (at the earliest) and originating in or around the Gobi Desert in what is now called China. In Earth time, that is the blink of an eye. *Y pestis* evolved from *Yersinia pseudotuberculosis*, which still exists around the world and causes mild diarrhea in humans. There is nothing mild about *Y pestis*.

Although it is primarily an infection of rodents, it incidentally infects humans by being injected via an insect—usually a bloodsucking flea—and has killed hundreds of millions of people across the globe. The history of *Yersinia pestis* shows how plagues have determined human history and will do so again.

YERSINIA PESTIS FROM THEN TO NOW

We know that all plague bacteria in the world today are descended from their ancestors that spread from Mongolia to Europe and from Europe back to China, to Yunnan province in the southwest to Hong Kong. From there, the bacteria voyaged round the world by steamship, in particular to the deserts of the southwestern United States where they chanced on an ecology that allowed them to persist.

Deoxyribonucleic acid (DNA) makes up the genes of all living things—fleas, hamsters, roses, *Y pestis*, elephants, butterflies, plankton, Brian, fish, *E. coli* . . . *all living things*—and is the blueprint for their replication. Paleobiology is a new science that studies DNA in ancient human remains and has resolved a number of historical controversies.

The earliest case of *Y pestis* infection recorded to date was found in the skeleton of a twenty-year-old female buried 4,900 years ago in what is now Sweden. She had DNA specific for *Y pestis* in her teeth pulp. Four thousand six hundred years ago in what is now called Estonia, a thirty-year-old woman from the Corded Ware culture lived and died on the shores of the Baltic Sea. Her skeletal remains were discovered in 1923, disinterred, and put in a museum. Returning to the skeleton ninety years later, researchers found *Y pestis* DNA in the pulp of her teeth. Similar evidence was found in six of 250 skeletal remains from locations that would later become Russia, France, and Armenia. These findings were of *Y pestis* without the *ymt* gene, necessary for the infection of fleas. These strains caused lethal pneumonia, but as they were not transmitted by fleas, they could not be said to cause bubonic plague.

But in 2018, *Y pestis* DNA was found in the tooth pulp of four out of nine skeletons in a kurgan or ceremonial grave in the Samara region of Russia. It was radiocarbon-dated to 3,800 years ago. These bacteria *did* possess the *ymt* gene. They are the earliest bacteria so far discovered that caused bubonic plague and push back the date of the first known human infection by a thousand years.

DNA analysis of the bacteria causing outbreaks of plague around the Caspian Sea and in East Asia in the last twenty years show an identical strain of *Y pestis* stemming from the Pontic-Caspian steppe, which is a vast grassland plain stretching from the Black Sea to the Caspian Sea, and from Romania to Kazakhstan. Horses first evolved on this plain. The earliest humans to domesticate and ride them were the Yamnaya pastoralists who four thousand years ago moved west along this corridor, taking the bubonic plague (and Indo-European languages) with them into Western Europe. This was the Bronze Age—human made tools, weapons, the potter's wheel, alcohol, legal codes, architecture, government, and early writing. Trade by ship on river and sea was gaining impetus. People traveled from China to the Mediterranean and back along the Silk Roads.

Homo sapiens is a wanderer. We wandered out of Africa to populate the world. Sometimes we were not wandering but running from war, famine, and disease. In this time, there were abrupt declines in Bronze Age culture around the eastern Mediterranean and the Pontic-Caspian steppe. There was the collapse of the Hittite empire, and while there are some tantalizing descriptions in the Torah and in Egyptian hieroglyphic writing, they do not reach the level of ironclad evidence for plague. From this point in history, there are two thousand years of bubonic plague to go before the first recorded-in-writing outbreak in 541 CE in Constantinople: the Justinian Plague.

There is the exception of Rufus of Ephesus. He was a physician practicing in 100 CE in modern-day Turkey and reported the writings of historians, whose works are now lost, that recounted an epidemic very like bubonic plague that killed a million people on the north coast of Africa in 300 BCE.

Despite his notations, it is customary to describe plague on Earth by citing the greatest documented European pandemics.

1. The Plague of Justinian from 541 CE–750 CE. Forty million died.
2. The European Black Death epidemics of 1348–1770. Fifty million died.
3. The Third Pandemic from 1896 to the present in which thirty million have died so far.

There is a fourth, often ignored in the West.

4. Bubonic plague in China. There have been epidemics from the 14th to the 19th century, and at least as many died as did in the Black Death in Europe. The disease continues there in small outbreaks.

This list of plague eruptions does not address—and it remains poorly understood—why the disease comes and goes. Justinian's plague lasted 200 years, and the Black Death continued intermittently in different parts of Europe for 450 years before being carried back to China.

PESTILENCE IN VENICE

Venice, like all seaports, is a focal point for plagues, and grievously has this city suffered from them. Between 1361 and 1528, the city experienced twenty-two outbreaks of bubonic plague, but the worst was yet to come. The plague of 1576–1577 killed a third of the population, after which the Basilica of the Redeemer, Il Redentore, was built to beseech God Almighty to show mercy on Venetians.

Venice had pioneered the concept of quarantine centuries earlier in 1377 during their control of Dubrovnik. Sailors, animals, and visitors from places where there was plague could not enter the city for *quarenta*, forty days, a biblical period. *Quarantine* is not the only Italian word associated with infectious diseases to pass into English. Sick patients were put on small plots of land in the lagoon, islands called *lazarettos*, or little houses of Lazarus who arose from the dead. There is hope. These islands were also used for quarantining, showing a remarkable level of early public health awareness particularly because it would be five hundred years before the germ theory of infection became established.

Plague was believed to be caused by miasmas, by *mal aria*, bad air. One infectious malady was called *influenza delle stelle*, the influence of the stars. In the 18th century, in a European pandemic, this astrology-based term spread northwards, and soon, in the English-speaking world, the disease became known as *influenza* and then *flu*.

In 1629, in Venice, out of a population of 140,000 people, 46,490 died of plague or smallpox, as both were raging. This devastation was known more widely as the Italian Plague of 1629–1631 as it ravaged northern Italy, including Milan.

In Venice, the Doge, Nicolo Contarini, died of an acute infection, but before he did, he ordered a solemn procession through the city for sixteen consecutive Saturdays bearing the miraculous icon of Madonna Nicopeia, and promised to build a basilica to the Virgin Mary after begging for her intercession. If Venice was delivered from the plague, there would be a ceremony of thanksgiving every year, forever. So, if you are in Venice on November 21, you may attend the service of gratitude at the Basilica of Santa Maria della Salute, Saint Mary of Health. These churches expressed faith and a conviction that the Blessed Virgin would plead their case and protect the Venetians from further plague.

Through the centuries, Venice was scourged by plague, smallpox, influenza, typhoid, typhus, and cholera. It is as much for these as any other reason that the power of Venice as a mercantile and political power declined.

Not one of the cities of Europe was spared the Black Death. Fifty million people amounted to over half the population. You may look up the name of any seaport active at that time to read how it was scourged: London, Marseille, Pisa, Florence, and Oslo along with Venice paid a particularly terrible toll. The agency of this force that could kill you and your family in a matter of days was to remain undiscovered for another 370 years.

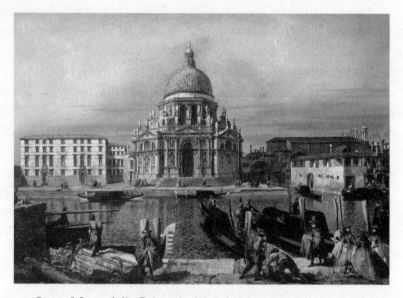

Santa Maria della Salute *by Michele Marieschi (1710–1744).*
The cause of the artist's death is lost to history.
Note his young age. Plague is most likely.

CRACKING THE CODE

Hong Kong, 1894. Doctor Alexandre Yersin, aged thirty-five, had been sent from Indochina, by the French Colonial Service, to determine the cause of a catastrophic outbreak of the bubonic plague in southwestern China. It took him ten days to do it.

Bubonic plague was infecting tens of thousands of people with a 70 percent mortality rate and was paralyzing the life of the city of Canton, now Guangzhou, ninety miles from the European colonies of Hong Kong and Macao.

Louis Pasteur, in 1850, had shown that bacteria, invisible without a microscope, were the cause of at least some feverish diseases. How many people in the world at that time believed this is hard to say. Surely a minority. Most of mankind felt that God or the gods were killing humans in large numbers to punish them for specified or unspecified sins. Alternative explanations were witchcraft, imbalance in Xi, scapegoating, and the position of the stars and the planets in the heavens. Whatever the cause, there was agreement that diseases were born on miasmas, mysterious clouds of ill health.

Alexandre Yersin had studied not only with Louis Pasteur but also with Robert Koch, who had discovered the bacteria that causes tuberculosis, and was fully educated in their methods. Yersin arrived in Hong Kong unheralded. The British Colonial Administration viewed this French citizen with suspicion, naturally, yet they gave him a permit to build a straw hut on the grounds of the Alice Memorial Hospital, the biggest in the city. He moved in with his microscope, other scientific paraphernalia, and a bed. He bribed British sailors in charge of the disposition of the dead to give him access to the corpses. Gloved, he would reach into coffins, brush aside the quicklime, and drain or excise buboes, the swollen lymph nodes that give the bubonic plague its name.

He wrote a clinical account of the plague.

Here are the symptoms and signs: Sudden appearance after an incubation of four and half to six days: there is severe fatigue and prostration. The patient suddenly succumbs to intense, often delirious high fever. On the first day a single bubo appears. 75 times out of 100, this bubo is found in the groin; 10 times out of 100 in the armpit; rarely on the neck or in other areas. The lymph node rapidly grows to the size of a hen's egg. Death comes 48 hours later, often earlier. When the patient is still alive after five or six days, the prognostic is better and the bubo softens; an operation can be performed to remove the pus.

Yersin reported a mortality rate of 95 percent in the hospitalized patients.

When he examined the pus, or "pulp," from excised buboes, he noted: *It always contains masses of short, stubby, rounded bacilli, which can be easily colored using aniline. The tips of the bacillus are more strongly dyed than the center, which gives it a transparent zone in the middle. Sometimes the bacilli look like they are surrounded by a capsule. They are always to be seen in the pulp of buboes, and sometimes in blood, although in much fewer numbers.*

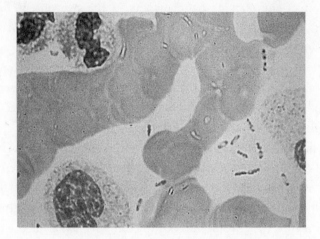

Yersinia pestis—a rod-shaped organism looking like a closed safety pin.

The Japanese scientist Kitasato Shibasaburo was also working in Hong Kong at the request of the Japanese government. He had also studied with Koch and had identified the same bacteria. There was debate as to who described it first. Thirty years later, Kitasato conceded that Yersin had primacy, and the organism is called *Yersinia pestis.*

Both Yersin and Kitasato injected the bacteria into rats, mice, and guinea pigs, inducing the disease in these animals. When the animals died, stained tissue and blood were positive for *Y pestis,* the bacterium they had injected.

Hong Kong, 1894

Chère Maman,

I'm sure you must be a little anxious to receive this letter, knowing I'm in a place one wouldn't exactly describe as a tourist destination!

The microbe looks like a little stick, longer than it is wide, and which is not difficult to stain. It kills mice and guinea pigs, which all display the lesions characteristic of the plague. It's always there; in my mind, there is no doubt.

Hong Kong is a very picturesque city, built on the slope of a sheer mountain 600 metres high, with houses staggered right up to the summit. The Chinese population numbers more than 200,000 souls. Fatality from Plague is very high: 95% of cases. Up until now only 3 Englishmen have been infected. I don't count the number of Portuguese; it's much higher. One of these days I'll try to take a little photograph of my straw hut with me standing in front and send it to you. I'm still keeping very well, aside from slight fatigue, because, as I'm on my own, I have to do everything myself.

I could tell you much more, but there are two bodies waiting for me, and the gentlemen seem in a hurry to get to the cemetery. Farewell, chère Maman, wash your hands after you've read my letter to avoid catching the plague!

Your son, affectionately, Alexandre

Yersin had discovered the cause of bubonic plague—the scourge that had killed hundreds of millions—within ten days of arriving in Hong Kong. It is brilliant and courageous work. As is always the case in science, one conclusion leads to another question. How does the microbe get into your bloodstream? He came close to answering this question, too.

I noticed that there were lots of dead flies in the laboratory where I performed my autopsies on animals. I ground down some of these flies into a broth and inoculated a guinea pig with it. The inoculation liquid contained a large quantity of bacilli similar in all respects to the plague bacillus, and the guinea pig died 48 hours later, displaying the lesions typical of the disease.

Even flies get the plague.

Alexandre Yersin left Hong Kong after a month of experiments, returning to Indochina, where he founded a medical school, continued his microbiological work, and received world recognition for his discovery. He lived to the age of eighty.

RODENT, INSECT, MAMMAL

Four years after Yersin had seen the Beast with his own eyes, Paul-Louis Simond, another Pasteurian, explained how the disease was transmitted. Simond was a British colonial officer assigned to Karachi in what is now Pakistan. A Hong Kong steamer had brought the plague to the Indian subcontinent where its effects were devastating and mirrored those of southern China. Ten million people died over the next four years. *Ten million!*

Through the study of patients, Simond noted that many in the early stage of infection had what looked like an insect bite. He manipulated dead black rats (*Rattus rattus*) to remove fleas in soapy water and quickly showed that these insects were packed with Yersin's bacteria.

Simond wrote, *I was fortunate enough to find a plague infected black rat in the home of a plague victim. I placed an uninfected rat in a cage separated from this rat by a grill through which only fleas could pass. I threw in many fleas I had harvested from a cat.*

The first rat died. Seven days later, the previously healthy rat died.

He observed, *I plunged the rat corpses into alcohol, and at autopsy there were abundant Yersin bacilli in the blood and organs. It is the flea that transmits the bacillus to man. Prophylactic measures against the Plague should therefore be directed towards rats, humans and fleas.*

The discoveries made by Yersin and Simond were rejected by the medical community. The idea that the bite of a flea who had bitten a rat transmitted disease was thought untenable by practicing clinicians. Pasteur's newfangled ideas about germs had not caught on. (They would not do so completely until the 1930s.) Doctors had been taught and believed in the miasma theory from the ancient Greek word meaning "pollution." Disease was transmitted by "bad air" or "night air." Moreover, it was widely and erroneously believed that rat fleas do not bite humans.

It was only after the work of the English Commission in India, published in 1908, that the transmission of Yersin's bacillus from rats to humans by fleas was established and universally accepted by the scientific community. It was also understood that patients with pneumonia could transmit the disease by coughing.

But is anything ever "universally accepted"?

As rats could not live in Northern Europe, where it i
can we explain plague outbreaks in Scandinavia or Icela
assuredly occurred?

The rat-flea-human model of Simond is not the only ... to explain
plague transmission. Other rodents, other insects—*Pediculus humanus* (the
human body louse) and *Pulex irritans* (the human as opposed to the rat
flea)—are known vectors, for example. The model is rodent-insect-mammal,
not just rat-flea-human. Over two hundred animals, predominantly mammals, may get infected with *Y pestis*. Sick people or sick animals can infect
others by coughing on them. In Colorado, the humans were infected by the
dog that had pneumonia. When people with pneumonic plague are crowded
together in insanitary cities, as they were throughout medieval Europe and
China, the disease will spread rapidly.

LET US CONSIDER THE FLEA

Xenopsylla cheopsis, the tropical rat flea, was first described by the entomol-
ogist Nathaniel Rothschild in 1909. Fleas are tiny, wingless insects with
bristles and spines that help them stick to the fur or hair of their hosts.
They are capable of jumping nonstop for days and have a life expectancy of
two to three months, but the adult form can lie dormant for up to a year.
On the Silk Roads from China to the Mediterranean, they likely hid in
furs, rolls of silk, or other traded items. There are at least 2,500 species of
flea, 80 of which transmit *Y pestis*.

They feed on blood at body temperature. When infected rats die, the
fleas leap off in search of a new host. They would prefer another rat. They
only bite humans if there is no other option. The blood of a dying rat (or
human) contains one hundred million *Y pestis* organisms per milliliter of
blood. The flea ingests about five thousand bacteria as it sucks in the blood.
They multiply in the flea's usually sterile midgut. The environment in the
gut of a flea is quite different from the infected animal's bloodstream. Temperature falls to the temperature of the flea. *Y pestis* has evolved a set of
genes that turn on to help it live in this new milieu. One of these is the
gene for a sticky protein. The sticky protein blocks the valve connecting

the esophagus to the midgut, leaving the flea hungry, so it bites repeatedly. In these futile feeding attempts, the sucked blood is pumped into the flea's esophagus where it dislodges bacteria, which are then regurgitated back into the wound of the original host or a new one. The fleas will then die of starvation.

Bubonic plague has caused the deaths of at least 300 million people. The death of one person is a tragedy. The saying goes on to say, the death of a million is a statistic. It isn't. It is a million tragedies. We can neither quantify nor encompass the human suffering that is the greater part of each plague. Emperors fell, empires collapsed, armies disintegrated, famine and more war followed. The history of mankind was changed forever because a bacteria secreted a sticky protein that blocked up the esophagus of a flea.

So, how do our four Coloradans and a dog acquire bubonic plague in 2014 in America? In 1894, rats bearing fleas containing *Y pestis* jumped aboard the steamships in Hong Kong and traveled around the world. By 1896, it had reached India. Soon there were new outbreaks of plague in the following places, all spread from Hong Kong by ship:

- Taiwan and Japan, 1896
- Bombay, India, 1896–1898
- Calcutta, India, 1898
- Madagascar, 1898
- Egypt, 1899
- Honolulu, Hawaii, and San Francisco, California, 1899
- Manchuria, China 1899
- Paraguay, 1899
- South Africa, 1899–1902
- Glasgow, Scotland, 1900
- Australia, 1900–1905
- Russian Empire/Soviet Union, 1900–present
- Fukien Province, China, 1901
- Siam, 1904
- Burma, 1905
- Suffolk, England 1906–1918
- Tunisia, 1907

- Bolivia and Brazil, 1908
- Trinidad, Venezuela, Peru, and Ecuador, 1908
- Cuba and Puerto Rico, 1912
- Pensacola, Florida, 1921

In December 1899, the plague had reached Honolulu. Authorities knew of the outbreak in Hong Kong, the plague harbor. All ships from Hong Kong flew a yellow flag, were inspected, and some were quarantined. Despite these precautions, You Chong, a twenty-year-old man in Honolulu's Chinatown, died on December 12. This was the first ever reported case of bubonic plague on the Hawaiian Islands and it was quickly followed by four more deaths. The disease spread into local rodents from ship rats and became endemic for the next thirty years.

Efforts to burn down a house in which plague had occurred "got out of control," and the whole of Chinatown, Honolulu, went up in flames. As news of these events reached San Francisco, it was received with great alarm by the Chinese community and indifference by everyone else. The *San Francisco Examiner* ran a headline: WHY SAN FRANCISCO IS PLAGUE PROOF.

The steamship *Australia* left its moorings in Honolulu and arrived at the Golden Gate on New Year's Day. She anchored at the quarantine station at Angel Island, was examined, and declared free of infection. The ship then moored near the sewage pipes discharging into the sea from Chinatown, San Francisco. *Rattus rattus,* the ship's rats, ran down the mooring ropes and into the sewers.

On March 6, 1900, Won Chut Xing, a forty-one-year-old lumber salesman, became the first human to die of bubonic plague on the North American continent. Chinese New Year had been celebrated a week before. By a cosmic irony, it was the Year of the Rat.

Plague exacerbated the prevailing anti-Chinese racism. "They" were already said to be responsible for smallpox and disseminating syphilis and were now harboring this new plague. Chinese Americans became simultaneously victim and scapegoat for pestilence in San Francisco.

Doctor Joseph J. Kinyoun was a quarantine officer and a federal public health official. He was another Pasteurian who had studied with the master in Paris. He aspirated pus from the lymph nodes of Won Chut Xing's corpse, stained it, and examined it under the microscope. They were there. Pink rods, stained at both ends, like an unopened safety pin. *Y pestis*, all right. He injected the pus into a monkey, a rat, and two guinea pigs. The Board of Health ordered that Chinatown be quarantined using a *cordon sanitaire* of thirty-two police officers to prohibit "Asians" from entering or leaving, while allowing white people to travel freely.

After three days, there were no new plague cases and the animals were still alive. Chinese Americans were threatening a lawsuit against the Board of Health asking for damages. Those who employed servants from Chinatown were chafing. Yet voices fell silent when, two days later, all three of the injected animals were dead. All stains were positive for *Y pestis*. Here was absolute proof of bubonic plague in San Francisco.

How did the city respond?

Not well. For the next two years, the media alleged that the Board of Health had lied and ridiculed Kinyoun and "his monkey." The governor of California, Henry Gage, suppressed evidence and openly lied about the situation. On June 14, after ten cases had been reported, the governor sent a manifesto to Secretary of State John Wyman stating, "There was no plague in the great and healthful city of San Francisco." Then, as always, plagues were bad for business. Governor Gage wasn't finished. He announced publicly that Surgeon Kinyoun had "imported vials of bubonic plague."

He wrote, *Could it be that some dead body of a Chinaman had innocently or otherwise received a postmortem inoculation in the lymphatic region by someone possessing the plague bacilli and that honest people were thereby deluded?*

Gage influenced the legislature of the United States to pass a joint resolution asking the president to remove Kinyoun from West Coast duty. Gage and the mayor kowtowed to the business community. They bartered the city's health for trade.

Kinyoun was reassigned to Oregon. Gage himself was undermined and lost the governorship in 1902. His successor quietly implemented the medical measures experts had been requesting, and the plague petered out. There had been 123 cases, 113 of whom died. An unappetizing gumbo of racism, ignorance, greed, and protectionism ushered *Y pestis* onto the

North American continent. So it goes. Yet only 113 people died. Recall that ten million died on the Indian subcontinent.

In 1906, San Francisco was struck by a devastating earthquake. As the city was rebuilding, the plague returned. The ruins of the earthquake made it easier for rats to breed. This time it was not centered in Chinatown. All the victims were Caucasian with cases in Oakland and Marin County. The political and health authorities reacted differently. There were 160 reported cases with 78 deaths, and for a second time the plague disappeared.

In 1908, the same year that the association between plague and fleas was established, a thirteen-year-old boy in Los Angeles died in three days from "pneumonia." Autopsy showed Yersin's bacteria everywhere in his body. In his yard were dead squirrels.

Plague in *Homo sapiens* living in the United States is rare. About ten cases a year have been diagnosed, and from records kept for the last twenty years, all are in the southwestern states. At Fort Collins, Colorado, the Centers for Disease Control and Prevention (CDC) monitors wildlife, controls fleas, and reports to the World Health Organization (WHO). If you should visit state parks out West, you will now understand the commonly seen warning signs of a red band running across the image of a squirrel. The sign says *Keep Wildlife Wild* and warns against approaching animals—particularly if they are sick or dead. Do not touch them. Do not pick them up.

There are seventy-six species of wild rodents in the United States. Ground squirrels, tree squirrels, marmots, chipmunks, and prairie dogs are infected by *Y pestis* with a very high mortality rate. Oddly enough, not all rodents suffer equally. There is great variation among species in response to plague. The California vole, deer mice, kangaroo rats, and grasshopper mice get little or no disease but act as a reservoir. Cats with bubonic plague almost all die. About a fifth of cases in the United States are due to cats contaminated by contact with wild rodents. Plague foci are often found in semiarid regions, like the western United States. Plague had flickered briefly in other American ports, but it firmly established itself in the West. Given the eighty species of flea, plus the other insects that can be infected with *Y pestis*, and the seventy-six rodent species, there is a very complex ecology at play.

An epidemic in animals is called an *epizootic*. Outbreaks in vulnerable species are explosive, with low resistance, high mortality, and rapid death. Such outbreaks increase plague transmission back to other susceptible rodents and mammals like coyotes, lynx, foxes, humans' pets, and human beings. It was good fortune indeed that the widespread slaughter suffered in southern China and on the Indian subcontinent did not repeat itself in California.

What happened to our Coloradan dog owner and the other three victims of the plague in 2014? The dog would have been infected by a flea or other insect vector that had gorged on blood from a wild type of rodent with the plague. The prairie dog is the most likely origin as epidemics are frequent among them. Autopsy of the dog showed pneumonia with *Y pestis* in the secretions. The dog's breath would have been teeming with bacteria, which would have been inhaled by Patient A., his friends, and the two veterinary technicians. This was the first report of a dog being a source of the plague in the United States and only the second ever published. The other was in China in 2009.

Of bacteria that cause disease, *Yersinia pestis* has been the greatest killer. It secretes toxins that disarm our innate immune system. The polymorphonuclear white blood cells that scavenge and engulf bacteria are paralyzed. It's as if they aren't there.

But not every infected person dies. Our Coloradan male was put on life support in the ICU. With intravenous antibiotics and supportive care, he survived after spending twenty-seven days there. The other three patients also recovered completely with antibiotic treatment.

All plague bacteria on the North American continent are descended from a single bacterium that made its way by rat, flea, and steamship from southern China to Hong Kong and then, via Honolulu, to California and through America's southwestern states. It is now ineradicable.

In July 2016, in New Mexico, a fifteen-year-old boy went to his doctor with fever and cough. He died two days later from plague. In 2020, an epidemic began in Madagascar that has killed two thousand humans so far.

The Third Pandemic has never ended. Shi Dao Nan, a poet who saw plague in 18th-century China and died from it at age twenty-seven, wrote:

Dead rats in the east
Dead rats in the west!
As if they were tigers,
Indeed are the people scared.
The hazy sun is covered by sombre clouds.
While three men are walking together,
Two drop dead within ten steps!
People die in the night,
Nobody dares weep over the dead!
The coming of the demon of pestilence
Suddenly makes the lamp go dim,
Then it is blown out,
Leaving man, ghost, and corpse in the dark room.
The crows caw incessantly,
The dogs howl bitterly!
Man and ghost are one,
There in the fields are crops,
To be reaped by none;
And the officials collect no tax!
I hope to ride on a fire dragon
To see the God and Goddess in heaven,
Begging them to spread heavenly milk,
And make the dead come to life again.

~Shi Dao Nan, 1765–1792

CHAPTER 4

....

RICE WATER: CHOLERA

Nigeria, 1972.

"I can't get the bloody IV catheter in!"

"You better hurry up."

A naked man of indeterminate age is lying on a wide canvas bed with a hole in the middle. Warm, watery, odorless stool is squirting over my sandals and socks. Cholera stool is like water. Sometimes you see white or pale-yellow bits in it, which is why it is called rice water stool. It is so thin you could read a newspaper through it. Should you have attempted this unlikely act with a Nigerian newspaper at that time, the headline would say, "No Cholera in Nigeria." This was read by all Nigerians to mean "Cholera definitely in Nigeria."

Lorries have been bringing in patients from all over Zaria, most from the old walled city but many from Tudan Wada, the mixed-tribe mercantile quarter. Some are brought in by car, a few walk in helped by friends, but the majority come in trucks. They are critically ill, about to become critically ill, or are dead. There is typically one dead person in each truck. Children are the most likely to be dead. Then the old. Confirming death is usually straightforward. But with cholera, an apparent corpse might take a sudden, deep breath. And I learned that breaking wind was not in itself a sign of life.

I touch the wrist of my patient, who is moribund. I can barely feel his pulse—about 130 beats a minute. Even on this hot summer's day on the Nigerian savannah, his extremities are cold. His leathery-looking skin had shrunk over his skull, his eyes were sunken in their hollow orbits, and his nails were blue. He is in the described-in-antiquity Blue Phase of Cholera. Which means, if I don't get the IV in, he's dead.

Cholera means *a gutter* in Greek. Or it may derive from *chole*, meaning "bile," as delineated in the theory of the four humours—according to the theory, the substances that make up the human body are black bile, yellow bile, blood, and phlegm. Hippocrates used the word *cholera* several times in his writings over two thousand years ago. But what he meant was diarrhea, of which there are many causes. *Trousse-galant* is used in France. It means "gallant kit." I don't know why cholera should be called gallant kit. It was also known as the Asiatic disease. No country except those on the Indian subcontinent had ever seen cholera before 1817. It existed there in epidemics for a long time, perhaps for two thousand years. In Sanskrit, it's *Visucika*. In Hindi, the word is *haiza*. In Bengali, *moryxy*. It may be a corruption of this word to call it *mordexin, merde-chi, mordeshi*. From which came *mort de chien*, used by the British in India, probably with an appalling accent, or *cramp* that's more stiff upper lip. In the 19th century, in which there were five global pandemics of cholera, names proliferated in accordance with theories of cause: *Trisplanchnasthenia, Hyperanthracis*. Terminological inexactitude has rendered impossible any accurate history of cholera before 1817. In several languages, the word *cholera* is used as an imprecation or insult. In Dutch, *Krijg de klere*—"Get Cholera and Die"; Yiddish, *Zol a Kholeira dir choppen*, or *A brannt dir in di Kishkes*—"May you get a burning in your intestines." Or it's an emphatic statement: *Naked Girls are Kholeira!* was the headline of a conservative Israeli newspaper article railing against nude beaches.

I'm going to cut the skin over his ankle vein to try and get the IV in there. It's not the most approved way, but at least I can see what I'm doing. The patient is taking deep, sighing breaths, *acidotic* breathing, with a kind of absolute apathy. His look says, "OK, everyone, I get it; I'm gone."

I need to work faster.

It's in.

"Just run it in, nurse, as fast as it will go. After he takes in two or three liters, then we'll take another look at him." Although the IV is now running, I am not convinced this man will survive. His brother is asking me desperate questions.

"Kwalara dokitah kwalara kwalara." There isn't an interpreter in sight.

"Hankali, hankali," I say. It's about all the Hausa, I know. It means "slowly." I learn the patient's name is Mohammed.

Earlier, I had put in an IV in a boy who subsequently died. He was twelve? Fourteen? His mother was ululating. Wailing. And the nurses were trying to lead her away from her son's deathbed. On the other hand, I'd seen another Blue Phase victim turn around yesterday after nine liters of intravenous normal saline. The first thing he asked for was pounded yam.

The first person to use intravenous fluid in history was Thomas Latta, an Edinburgh physician in 1832, in a patient with cholera.

I at length resolved to throw the fluid immediately into the circulation. The first subject of experiment was an aged female. She had apparently reached the last moments of her earthly existence, and now nothing could injure her—indeed, so entirely was she reduced, that I feared I should be unable to get my apparatus ready ere she expired. Having inserted a tube into the basilic vein, cautiously—anxiously, I watched the effects; ounce after ounce was injected, but no visible change was produced. Still persevering, I thought she began to breathe less labouriously, soon the sharpened features, and sunken eye, and fallen jaw, pale and cold, bearing the manifest impress of death's signet, began to glow with returning animation; the pulse, which had long ceased, returned to the wrist; at first small and quick, by degrees it became more and more distinct . . . and in the short space of half an hour, when six pints had been injected, she expressed in a firm voice that she was free from all uneasiness, actually became jocular.

A hundred and seventy years later, I have a patient in the same situation. Certainly, he has death's signet, but I hope he has the same recovery. For a hundred and fifty years we have known what causes cholera and how to stop it, yet it persists. Why?

CHOLERA AND JOHN SNOW

William Sproat, a dockworker from Sunderland, became the first man to die on British soil from cholera during the Second Pandemic. In that year, 1832, 52,000 others followed. In a Yorkshire mining village, John Snow, an eighteen-year-old assistant surgeon, recorded every patient, every death, and every recovery in an exercise book on the cover of which he had written CHOLERA in capital letters with a black pencil. He noted that miners and their families suffered more than other occupations, also observing that there were no privies in the pits and that miners ate with unwashed hands. He noted that women and children acquired the disease a day or two after the men.

John Snow has strong views. He is a vegetarian and a teetotaler. As a physician, he believes that good food and clean water are essential for health. He has developed a habit that will last a lifetime—he writes his medical views and publishes them.

In 1836, the young Yorkshireman decides to further his career in London. He walks the two hundred miles to the city. He passes all his exams and becomes interested in the use of ether and chloroform for general anesthesia. He devises an apparatus and a mask to administer them. He is summoned by an enthusiastic Prince Albert to administer chloroform to Queen Victoria during the birth of her last two children, Prince Leopold and Princess Beatrice. All goes well. These are dizzying heights for this modest man of modest origins. Surely, he has made it! He can become a society physician, Anaesthetist to the Court! He isn't interested. If this were all we knew of Dr. Snow, it would be a lot. It was said of him that "He made the Art of Anaesthesia a Science."

He never married. He is considered taciturn and emotionally flat. He lives on the prosperous side of Regent Street, ten minutes' walk from his busy clinic in Soho, one of London's most densely populated areas—in other words, a crowded slum. At night he writes prolifically or does further research with his gases on birds or mice kept in his living room. He works hard every day to prove his assertions. He was a singular man.

In 1834, cholera tapered off and disappeared in the British Isles. Londoners forgot about it. They already had to live with tuberculosis, scarlet fever, diphtheria, rheumatic fever, life expectancy of forty, grinding poverty, hunger, and a high infant mortality. Men worked as bone pickers, rag gatherers, dredgermen, mudlarks, bunters, shoremen, eel skinners, and cats' meats men. Many came in intimate contact with feces. What's a little cholera? It is forgotten except by the voiceless poor, who lost those they loved and who were often scapegoated for causing the disease.

John Snow did not forget.

When the Third Pandemic returned to the British Isles in 1848, killing fifty thousand in London alone, Snow published his treatise *On the Mode of Communication of Cholera* (1849). He proposed that cholera is transmitted by humans, and new infections are seeded by individuals arriving from places where the disease is prevalent. He stated that the disease was localized in the intestines and was caused by drinking water contaminated by feces.

Although it was a well-reasoned argument, not to mention true, few agreed with him. Of those in a position to do something about it, none agreed. John Snow was a contagionist. The medical establishment thought little of them. In a survey of American physicians at the time, fewer than 5 percent accepted contagion as a cause for disease. Some of Snow's colleagues thought it was due to lack of ozone, others that it was caused by telluric, which is a poison emitted from the earth. Senior ministers of the Church of England would preach that the disease had been sent by Divine Providence to scourge the populace for their sins, particularly drunkenness and debauchery.

Yet the dominant explanation for all diseases, and cholera in particular, was miasma. "All smell is disease," said Edwin Chadwick, chairman of the General Board of Health, to a parliamentary committee set up to investigate the problem of sewage. The disease was seen in places out of which foul smells were emerging. The odor, therefore, was the cause.

Snow, meanwhile, continued his painstaking review of the records and showed that cholera was more frequent in those Londoners who got their water from a company that drew it directly out of the Thames at Hungerford Bridge than in those who took water further upstream from Thames Ditton.

On Monday, August 28, 1854, a baby, family name of Lewis, residing at 40 Broad Street, fell ill with vomiting and diarrhea. This child's illness caused small interest to the urban uproar of Victorian Soho. In the area were a workhouse, a brewery, and a factory that made percussion caps for rifles. It was hot. The new standardizing scale of temperature measurement, Fahrenheit, said it was ninety degrees for three days in a row. By coincidence, it was just in this part of town that John Snow's clinic was situated.

The Soho epidemic started on a Sunday night, but it was two more days before people began to manifest cholera. The Lewis baby was still ill. Other people in the area were falling sick. By Thursday morning, hundreds were seized. Entire families were infected, ailing in dark, suffocating rooms. Friday, September 1, the first deaths are reported. There is cholera elsewhere in London, but it is sparse.

A year later, looking back, John Snow writes in his book *On Cholera*,

> *The mortality in this limited area probably equals any that was ever caused in this country, even by the plague; and it was much more sudden as the greater number of cases terminated in a few hours. The mortality would undoubtedly have been much greater had it not been for the flight of the population . . . in less than six days from the commencement of the outbreak, the most afflicted streets were deserted by more than three quarters of their inhabitants.*

Late on the evening of September 1, he walks across Regent Street from his home on Sackville Street, Mayfair, along Carnaby Street to Broad Street. He wants to examine the area in tranquility and to collect samples from the pump to examine under his microscope. That day he had attended three cases of undoubted cholera surrounded by the turmoil of death. He walks toward the pump from Cambridge Street. It's an intuition. He suspects the pump immediately. Now, he needs to collect the evidence. There is a hearse on the street. Overall, it is quiet and deserted. Yellow flags are flying at ten-yard intervals to warn of pestilence. A gentleman approaches him.

"Excuse me, sir, I think we have met before." He is thirtyish.

"Dr. John Snow."

"Ah, yes. I am Henry Whitehead, the Reverend Henry Whitehead."

"Curate at St. Luke's, I think."

"Precisely, sir. What have you learned, sir, from this pestilential outbreak?"

"Nothing so far. I am looking at the pump."

"These foul miasmas, sir. They stem from poverty and too many people crammed together. Poor ventilation is at the root of it."

John Snow operates the pump handle. He pulls a glass medicine bottle from his coat pocket and catches some of the water. He holds it up to the gaslight.

"It looks clear, but I will need to examine it further." He corks and pockets it.

The Reverend Whitehead catches a few drops in his hands and drinks.

"For God's sake, man. Don't drink that water!"

He pushes Whitehead's hands away.

"Just a little thirst, Doctor."

The reverend makes to collect some more.

"Do not drink the water!"

"What are you saying, man?"

"I am saying, oblige me, sir, and do not drink water from that pump."

"Very well. You are a contagionist, I see."

"I am, Reverend."

"I am not a medical man, Dr. Snow, but I feel that the atmosphere all over the world is at this time favorable to the production of the most formidable plagues."

"Tomorrow, Mr. Whitehead, I will go to the Registry Office to find the names of the people who have died and then I shall go to those households and obtain what information I can. And for now, sir, I bid you good night."

The Reverend Henry Whitehead's pastoral duties include visiting the houses of the sick and dying. In a large house on the corner, Green Court, all twelve died. He sees the devastating results of the epidemic.

We can imagine him walking along streets white and milky from the antiseptic chloride of lime, the air sharp with its acrid odor. Men and women are dressed in mourning. The only topic of conversation is the pestilence. Rumors spread that placing sewage conduits near Golden Square had disturbed the four thousand corpses buried there in 1653, dead from bubonic plague, and thus caused the epidemic. So many were dead this day of cholera that coffins were placed on top of hearses or on death carts. Parochial handbills were plastered everywhere, and yellow flags flew. Shopkeepers told how they had spoken to a perfectly healthy person that morning who was dead by sundown.

Snow made detailed enquiries into each of the eighty-nine fatal cases that had occurred so far. Nearly all the deaths had taken place within a short distance of the pump. At least sixty-nine of those who died had drunk water from it. A committee of the guardians of St. James's Parish listened to Dr. Snow and agreed to remove the pump handle. On September 8, nine days into the outbreak, the pump handle was removed.

ZARIA, NIGERIA, 1972

There are more lorries being unloaded in casualty. I put my sandals and socks in the incineration bin. There are ten million bacteria per cc—I put boots on, wash my hands, and go back for a second round. The management of cholera is pretty straightforward—get the IV in. If they are not apathetic, or blue, and not vomiting, give them fluid by mouth. All they can drink.

At lunch, Jack Slocombe, Professor of Tropical Medicine at the London School of Hygiene and Tropical Medicine, is visiting and giving us a lecture. We are having bananas and bottled water.

He says, "The Delta of the Ganges is the home of cholera. It spread from there across all the continents of the world in the 19th century. Everywhere. And in India, Bangladesh, Indonesia, and we fear, now, sub-Saharan Africa, it has become endemic. It spreads fast. The waves out of India were known as the Six Pandemics. There were two in the first half of the nineteenth, three in the second half, and one at the beginning of the twentieth that, more or less, dwindled away by 1945. Then there came a lull of a few years. You are now in the Seventh. It started in earnest two years ago hitting Africa first in Guinea. It is caused by *Vibrio cholera type 01, biotype El Tor.*"

"Hey," shouts out my colleague McTavish, "I thought El Tor was just a mild diarrhea?"

"Questions at the end, please," says the moderator.

"No, it's OK," says Slocombe. "McTavish and I are old friends. You're right in a sense, McTavish. Let me answer it in this way. It is milder. That is, it kills its victims more slowly, and this gives patients the opportunity to walk and disseminate the disease. It also has the luxury of travel by air, train, and automobile more quickly than classic cholera ever could. But it is cholera, all right."

"Our patients seem to have classic cholera, not some mild attack of the runs."

"Well, we haven't identified your microorganism yet, and it's true that the CFRs [Case Fatality Rates] are lower with El Tor, but it is still a lethal process. I am betting that this is a variety of the El Tor strain, perhaps with a local modification. To continue, I want to get on to treatment."

McTavish sits, tight lipped.

"I want to discuss Oral Replacement Therapy, ORT. We have two studies, one from Cash and Nallin working in Bangladesh. They had great success with oral rehydration. The key thing is that glucose stimulates reabsorption of sodium in the small bowel. To repeat, it is the concentration of glucose that drives sodium, and with it, water back into the circulation. Second, and this is information I have only just received—it is unpublished, coming out in the *Journal* next month—of a truly remarkable result by a man called Dilip Mahalanabis. He is working in a refugee camp of thirty-five thousand in India on the border with Bangladesh. There are hundreds more pouring in each day. Naturally, there is cholera. So, he has lorries running in every couple of days from Calcutta with inexpensive, prepackaged salt-glucose powder. They treated three thousand people in three weeks. His Case Fatality Rate was 3.6 percent."

McTavish is glaring. He looks as if he might explode. This isn't his first epidemic. Everyone knows he treated cholera in Afghanistan. McTavish is a legend.

Slocombe continues, "Under these circumstances, 3.6 percent is fantastically good. So, with ORT, have we just rediscovered the obvious? The treatment of cholera is water and glucose by mouth."

McTavish explodes. "Do you really think that two or three cups of fruit juice are going to save the lives of our patients? What about those two chaps you saw this morning? Do you think they would get better without intravenous fluid? I mean, you give them water, it goes straight though. Well, doesn't it?"

"Oh no," said the professor. "Don't misunderstand me. Patients in shock should continue to have intravenous fluid. What fluids are you giving them?"

"Normal saline, isotonic. I think that's what you need when your patient is lying there without a pulse, blue around the gills and . . ."

"Yes, no. Listen, McTavish, I agree. Everyone agrees. You still need an IV for patients in shock. You should probably give them glucose as well. And potassium. On physiological principles. Evidence suggests that the sooner you start treating patients with oral therapy containing glucose, salt, and potassium, the fewer you are going to see going into shock."

McTavish was going into shock. "I've read Chatterji." He is almost shouting. "And Awqati, and what about Phillips? He showed you have to give IV fluids." He *is* shouting. He sits down.

Methodically, the professor presses on. "So, I am suggesting that in your sick patients, not those in shock, you give them oral therapy. I have a recipe: twenty grams of glucose, three and a half grams of sodium chloride, one and a half grams of potassium chloride, half a gram of sodium bicarbonate dissolved in a liter of water."

"How about antibiotics?" asks a voice from the back of the room.

A few more questions, then it's back to work. I go with my pediatrician chum Bill Sherman. I do not envy him. With patients so small, scalp vein needles are not easy to place. I return to see how my patients are getting on. Mohammed, the man with the IV in his ankle, has a stronger pulse. Its rate is down to 110 beats per minute. He still seems profoundly apathetic, but there is some response. He does sort of twitch his legs if you talk loudly at him.

At about five thirty, the sun drops quickly below the horizon. Mohammed continues to improve. He's not asking for pounded yam yet, but his blood pressure is up. He is passing urine, and his pulse is down to ninety beats per minute. He still looks completely bewildered and isn't moving much.

"Mohammed," I shout. "Mohammed, Ina ka je?"

His head jerks. He says nothing.

I wake in the night and have a little diarrhea. In a pit latrine. I don't know where it goes from there. If anywhere. There is a scorpion looking at me as I relax. It scuttles away. I think, *What if I'm having the famous premonitory diarrhea of cholera?* Maybe I'm having cholera itself, a mild go-round. Could be. Many people get infected and have little or no diarrhea. They carry it around for a week or two, though, which spreads it to others. Overall, I'm not too worried. If I have cholera, I will survive. Those who get to the hospital survive; those who don't, die. In the morning, I feel fine. No nausea, no vomiting. No abdominal pain. No leg spasms. Next morning, I drink a carefully made cup of tea, then off to work in my orange Beetle.

Mohammed had recovered overnight. Another bloody miracle. He is sitting up.

"Sannu, Mohammed."

"Sannu, Likita."

His demeanor suggests he has been caught out in a willful prank. "Okay, then, fair enough," he seems to say. "I had cholera; it's a fair cop." He is bashfully drinking a cup of water.

"Any diarrhea?"

"No, no any. Humdillah."

"I think we can take that needle out now."

Professor Jack Slocombe wants to make rounds with me for an hour before leaving for Kano and his flight back to London. I've been excused from cholera duty today. He wants to see some "everyday" tropical disease to remind him of the year he had worked in Bangkok. We see typhoid; purulent pericarditis; probable tuberculosis; *Schistosomiasis mansoni* with gastrointestinal bleed; guinea worm, aka dracunculiasis with acute arthritis; and severe "algid" malaria.

As we make the rounds, I say, "Professor, I have a question that has been bothering me."

"Yes," he responds cautiously.

"Why is the Delta of the Ganges the home of cholera?"

"Good question. Don't know. Where is the pump handle, so to speak? Sure, they are poor and crowded together and may not have access to clean drinking water. But why it should start there and spread all over the world ... We are entering the global era of infectious diseases, you know."

"Yes, I'm sure that's true. Interesting, though, isn't it? Why the Delta of the Ganges?"

"Well, look, look me up next time you are in London. We can go to John Snow's pub and discuss it there."

"He has a pub named after him?"

"Of course. The highest accolade the British can bestow on an illustrious son. It's in the same spot as it was in 1855. Different name then. Changed a bit, I expect. But they have a visitor's book. People visit from all over the world. Peking, Los Angeles, Birmingham. It's worth a visit just to look at that book. Beer's not bad either. But, of course, John Snow was a teetotaler. Not sure if he'd approve."

"Well, I'm prepared to celebrate the man. And you can't drink the water on Broad Street."

LONDON, 1854

John Snow and the removal of the Broad Street pump handle is a gesture that resonates to this day. Here begins public health. Here begins the science of epidemiology. It is a turning point in the history of medicine. Although it has been romanticized and simplified as you might expect, there are three points to be made.

The first is that the removal of the pump handle did not immediately stop the epidemic. It was declining anyway.

The second is that the medical establishment poured scorn on Dr. Snow's idea and rejected it to a man. Benjamin Hall, president of the General Board of Health, expressed open disbelief. Edwin Chadwick, sanitary commissioner of London, said it was illogical. The *Lancet* said, "In riding his hobby very hard, he has fallen down through a gully-hole and has never since been able to get out again. Has he any facts to show in proof? No!" The *Lancet* instead blamed cholera on "the atmosphere or its concomitant imponderable agents." "Concomitant imponderable"—what an excellent meaningless phrase!

The third is that the Reverend Henry Whitehead deserves equal credit with Dr. John Snow in solving the riddle of the Broad Street cholera epidemic in which, all told, five hundred people died in a two-week period, most of them living within 250 yards of the Broad Street pump.

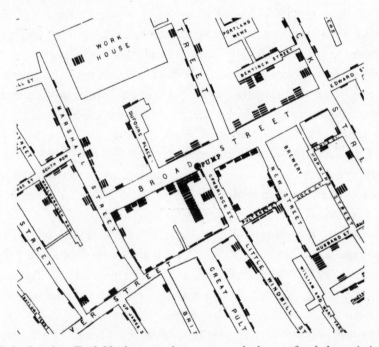

Soho London. Each black rectangle represents the house of a cholera victim. Note how they cluster round the pump.

The Committee of St. James Vestry started its own enquiry. Both Snow and Whitehead were conscripted to write reports. In January 1855, Snow's book on cholera was published. He gave a copy to Whitehead, who wrote him a letter back detailing his objections to the hypothesis— what he called the *Snovian* hypothesis. He went to work himself, certain he could prove Snow wrong. He visited and/or revisited household after household, sometimes several times, to confirm details. His report was forty-two pages long and was submitted to the committee in June 1855.

Slowly and reluctantly at first, by an analysis of the evidence, Whitehead came around to Snow's point of view. Of the residents in the area, only two of those with cholera had not drunk water from the pump. Of twenty-eight nonresidents with cholera, twenty-four worked in factories where the pump water was in constant use. Of those who did not get cholera, residents and nonresidents, twenty-nine drank the pump water; 279 did not. There were also individual cases who did not live in the area. The most crucial was the Widow of Hampstead, whose husband had owned the percussion cap factory. She loved Broad Street pump water and had her sons bring her two bottles daily. Both she and her niece, who also drank the water, acquired cholera and succumbed. Whitehead found the sons, who both confirmed that they had taken the water to Hampstead. She drank the water on Thursday, acquired cholera on Friday, and died on Saturday. No other case of cholera was noted in Hampstead.

At the Lion Brewery on Broad Street, none of the eighty employees had cholera. They drank water from their independent well. At the workhouse round the corner on Poland Street, no one died. They took their water from the Poland Street pump.

Reviewing the registry, Whitehead's eye catches a date of death. The Lewis baby. Sick from the thirtieth, died four days later. The father, a policeman, one of the new Peelers, named for police force founder Sir Robert Peel, had acquired cholera five days after his infant daughter. He lived an unusually long eleven days before death.

The reverend revisits the grieving widow at 40 Broad Street. She tells him how she steeped the unclean napkins (diapers) in buckets and then threw the watery contents into the cesspit at the front of the house. Whitehead summons a surveyor, Jehoshaphat York, whose investigation finds the cesspit less than three feet from the well and eight feet above it. The bricks were rotten, and the swampy soil was saturated with human filth. The contents of the cesspit were seeping into the Broad Street well.

The widow threw her husband's diarrheal output and the water she washed his clothes with in the same cesspit at the front of the house, next to the pump. By then, however, the handle had been removed. Being in such close contact with her child and husband, how did the young woman survive?

Come to think of it, how did Snow and Whitehead survive? They must have been aware of the risk they were running by being in close contact with sick and dying patients. Yet nowhere in their writing is there the slightest sense of anxiety, caution, or dread.

As Whitehead came to see that Snow was right, a friendship developed between these two abstemious and celibate men. They may be imagined, the Yorkshireman and the man of Kent sitting in the front parlor drinking tea. Entirely Victorian. When the talk turns to cholera, they will be wondering when it will be a thing of the past. The trouble is, cholera is still not a thing of the past.

Few in London would have known that there was an outbreak of cholera in Florence in 1854. Filippo Pacini, pathologist, found the comma-shaped bacteria when looking at the mucosa of the intestines of a victim at autopsy. He published his findings. They were ignored until thirty years after his death. Pacini insisted cholera was contagious and caused by the comma-shaped bacteria. He was the first human to see it. He died in poverty and obscurity. Robert Koch, unaware of Pacini's work, rediscovered the bacillus in 1884. He managed to grow the organism in nutrient broth with salt.

It was not until the beginning of the 20th century that the miasma theory was put to rest. John Snow died of "apoplexy," or stroke, at the age of forty-five in 1858. This premature death has been attributed to chronic renal failure caused by his self-experimentation with anesthetic agents. His obituary in the *Lancet* read, "This well-known physician died at noon on the 16th instant, at his house in Sackville street from an attack of apoplexy. His researches on chloroform and other anesthetics were appreciated by the profession."

That was it.

In 2013, 155 years later, the *Lancet* apologized to the memory of the man who established epidemiology.

THE GREAT STINK

Then came an event to make even Parliament act: the Great Stink. In Shakespeare's day, the population of London, the largest city in the world, was two hundred thousand, a huge number. Two hundred and forty-two years after the poet's death, it was two million. By the end of the 19th century, it would be six million.

In June 1858, the smell off the river was so vile that it sent parliamentarians running with handkerchiefs pressed to their noses. Benjamin Disraeli was running with them, loudly cursing "Stygian Pools." Parliament was closed down. The press, which meant the *Times*, the *Illustrated London News*, the *Observer*, and *Punch*, were merciless. They railed against politicians. The prevailing messages was—now that the stench has closed them down, perhaps these lazy good-for-nothings will do something about it. *Whoso once inhales the stink*, wrote one journalist, *can never forget it and can count himself lucky if he lives to remember it.*

One odd thing. In spite of the increase in smell, there was no increase in cholera. John Snow, who died that year, might have left the mandarins a last word, something he had said at a meeting years before. "We must do away with that form of liberty to which some communities cling, the sacred power to poison to death not only themselves but their neighbours."

Enter Joseph Bazalgette, engineer. He was invited to clean the largest city in the world of pestilence and filth. He was to solve man's historic struggle with excrement. He had a partner in this venture. James Newland had started the construction of the world's first integrated sewer system in Liverpool ten years before. Both men had vision and engineering genius, and worked hard.

Bazalgette planned and supervised the construction of 82 miles of main sewers and 1,100 miles of street sewers with major pumping stations to bypass the city, dumping into the Thames Estuary on the high ebbing tide.

On the 27th of June in 1866, the last British cholera epidemic to date swept through London. Approximately six thousand people died. They were confined to the East End of London where Bazalgette's system of sewers was not yet in place. Ninety-three percent of the deaths were in an area served by the East London Water Company. Physician William Farr was sent to investigate. This ardent believer in miasma theory, and one who had dismissed John Snow's ideas, had at last seen the light. Both Farr and the *Lancet* now accepted contagion theory.

Not only was the 1866 epidemic the end of cholera in London; it was also the end of typhoid—except for occasional imported cases, some of which came from the massive epidemic in Hamburg in 1892.

As much as Sir Christopher Wren is responsible for the London that exists above the horizon, Sir Joseph Bazalgette takes equal credit for the structures below. One is as necessary and beautiful as the other. There is a small monument to him under Charing Cross Railway Bridge. It has been said that he saved more lives than any single Victorian public official.

Of the great sewer that runs beneath, Londoners know, as a rule, nothing. The Registrar General could tell them that its existence has added twenty years to their chance of life.

~the *Times*

THE ORIGIN OF CHOLERA

Vibrio cholerae are descendants of a bacteria that first appeared 670 million years ago. It multiplies every seventeen minutes. In recent times—that is, over the last million years or so—it has lived in estuarine and brackish water. It is found in all the shores and estuaries of the world, even in places, such as Iceland, which have never had a single case of the disease. There are two hundred different serotypes, and it is one of the most abundant bacterial families. *Vibrio cholera serotypes O1* and *O139* (the cause of current cholera in China) are the only strains among many *vibrio* strains that cause the disease. El Tor is a variant of O1. *El Tor* is the Arabic word for Mount Sinai and is named after an outbreak on the Sinai Peninsula in 1905. It is the cause of the Seventh Pandemic, spanning the 1960s to the present. It looks like a swimming peanut. The DNA of the bacteria is made of four million base pairs arranged in two chromosomes. Both chromosomes were sequenced in 2000.

After all that has been said so far, it may be surprising to hear that cholera is not caused by the bacteria *Vibrio cholerae*. It is caused by a toxin produced by a virus that is constrained to live in the bacteria. Sambhu Nath De, a Bangladeshi scientist, discovered the toxin in 1959. The toxin is a protein with two parts, A and B. Protein part A attaches to the cells of the small bowel, and part B is drawn into them where it leads to the excretion of chloride from the cell. Think of it like this. We are 70 percent water, held in place by membranes. The toxin rips those membranes open and all your water falls out. However, not everyone infected gets the disease, but they can certainly carry the organism with them to another place. These are the asymptomatic carriers of cholera.

To answer the question I posed to Professor Jack Slocombe, there are a number of reasons that the Delta of the Ganges is the home of cholera:

1. **Human elements**

   To acquire cholera, you must drink water or eat food, most often seafood, contaminated with *Vibrio cholerae*. You need to take in between 10^2 and 10^6 bacteria. *Vibrio cholerae* causes diarrhea containing 10^8 bacteria—that's a hundred million per gram of feces. Contamination of the water supply is the usual way that cholera is spread, as was seen in the case of the Broad Street epidemic. You may also acquire cholera by the feco-oral route, if you are in close contact with a person in the throes of infection, but this is less common. You are more likely to catch it if you have reduced or no stomach acid from taking antacids or from having disease that lowers stomach acid and if you are malnourished or have impaired immunity. You are more likely to die if you are a child, as dehydration is more rapid than in an adult. Pregnant women are also vulnerable and fetal death is common. If you have blood group O, you are at greater risk of death—up to eight times more likely—the reason is unknown. The lowest incidence in the world of this blood group is in the Delta of the Ganges.

   Kolkata in India and Dhaka in Bangladesh are built on the largest estuary delta in the world, the confluence of the Ganges River, the Brahmaputra River, and the Bay of Bengal. Four hundred million people live in the Ganges River Basin, making it one of the most densely populated regions on Earth. Poverty and overcrowding are widespread, and sanitation is primitive. Cholera occurs year-round in Bangladesh with well-described peaks of disease in the spring and fall, before and after the monsoon. This implies that other factors are at play.

2. **Bacterial elements**

Estuarine waterways are a seething mass of biodiversity. At the microscopic end, DNA is shared or transferred among viruses, bacteria, and plankton such as diatoms and protozoans, as well as small crustaceans and the eggs and larval stages of larger animals. They eat each other, strike random biochemical survival bargains, and are more likely to be parasites and symbionts than not, intermingling at a dizzying level of complexity, evolving, and counter-evolving. *Vibrio* live and flourish in the estuarine waters of the Ganges because of the relationship they have with one of the world's most prevalent planktons, the copepod. Numerous *Vibrio* cling to its shell and its intestinal cells. This benefits them in times of restricted resources. They become dormant and tolerate temperatures, levels of acidity, and salinity that they never could tolerate in an independent state. It may protect them from stomach acid when copepods are eaten. It is the bacteria's relationship with the copepod that accounts for its wide dispersal in the oceans. When the number of copepods is high, the chance of cholera is high. What good is all this knowledge to the men and particularly the women of Bangladesh who carry and handle the water? Sieving water removes plankton. If you sieve your drinking water through a folded cloth, it will reduce the incidence of cholera by 50 percent.

3. **Environmental elements**

The Delta of the Ganges is tropical, wet, and prone to cyclones and flooding. With global warming, the risk of rising sea levels is critically appreciated. Cholera admissions to hospitals correlate with sea surface temperature, salinity, river level, and the amount of rain.

Professor Rita Colwell is a microbiological scientist who has dedicated her life to the study of cholera, and she has joined the immortals. She showed that *Vibrio cholerae* lived in the sea before man began polluting it, that it is closely associated with copepods, and she outlined the environmental factors that make cholera more likely. She was able to measure such variables as water level, sea surface temperature, and chlorophyll levels in the sea (which correlates with the amount of copepod) and plot them with satellite photography. This is our modern map of the Broad Street Pump.

Taking these elements all together, a perfect storm of risks, you can see why cholera found a home in the Delta of the Ganges, and find clues as to why this plague persists.

Cholera has not gone from the world. Since 2016, an outbreak of cholera in Yemen has been augmented by war and famine with lack of medical support. As of January 2020, there have been over 2,300,000 estimated cases in this outbreak, making it the most severe cholera epidemic ever recorded.

CHAPTER 5

....

OF LICE AND MEN: TYPHUS

F ive hundred million years ago, a bacteria called *Pelagibacter ubique* was flourishing—and still is. It is the most prevalent bacteria in the oceans, and, probably, the world. It is also one of the smallest, and it replicates slowly, once every twenty-four hours. At some point, a sub-species of this organism began to live in protists, or single-celled organisms, to the benefit of both.

A hundred and fifty million years ago, a group of these symbiotic bacteria, called the *Rickettsiae*, coalesced. They lived, and still live, in insects. They are transmitted through the ovary into the young of the insect they are infecting. They also infect plants. They are injected by insect bite into vertebrates, where they cause a feverish illness with a number of consequences, including death.

Three hundred thousand years ago, *Homo sapiens* appeared on the planet. *Rickettsial* infections must have afflicted them. So far, there is no evidence of this.

In 430 BCE, an epidemic befell the city of Athens as recorded by Thucydides. This was probably typhus, although in 1935, Hans Zinsser, the author of *Rats, Lice and History*, thought it was smallpox. Typhus is caused by a *rickettsial* organism.

In 1489, in the siege of Baza, the army of Don Ferdinand of Aragon suffered serious losses from a "malignant spotted fever." He lost three thousand men in battle and 17,000 to an infection characterized by severe headache, a rash, conjunctivitis, mental confusion, and delirium followed by death.

Typhus, the most severe of all *rickettsial* infections, is named for a Greek word, *tûphos*, meaning "cloud" or "fog," and refers to delirium. This same disease occurred in Mexico in 1545 and throughout Europe in the 16th century. In both locations, there were extensive and continuing wars leading to overcrowding of soldiers in unsanitary conditions.

In 1618, the Thirty Years' War spread the pestilence throughout Europe from Amsterdam to Montpelier to Berlin. "Spreading the pestilence" sounds neat and tidy, but what it led to was deserted cities with corpses decomposing in the streets.

From 1625 on, in the prisons and ships of England, men were dying of "gaol [jail] fever" and "ship fever." Both settings are ideal for typhus—close quarters and limited sanitation. Typhus is transmitted by the body louse, which lives and breeds in dirty clothing or bedding. The unlucky louse will usually die in seven days, sick itself from infection, but its feces are thick with bacteria. The feces are the source of the infection, and scratching the louse bite (not the bite of the louse itself) is what spreads typhus. It can also be caught by inhaling dried louse feces or rubbing them in the eyes. Humans are a reservoir for the bacteria, as is our old friend the black rat.

Being jailed at that time was a risk for death from typhus. Society at large did not mind this very much until the Black Assizes at Oxford in 1577. Rowland Jenkes, a saucy, foul-mouthed bookseller being tried for scandalous words against the Queen, was brought before the court.

"...a foul air arose from the prisoners taken out of a noisome Gaol ..."

The judges, the jury, witnesses, "every person except the prisoners, and they alone were not injured by it," grew sick. My Lords the Chief Baron of the Exchequer and the High Sheriff died, likely from having inhaled dried louse feces. The infection spread into the city, and about three hundred more deaths followed. Jenkes had his ears cut off but went on to live a long, earless life.

The Marshalsea and the Fleet in London were typical jails of the land. As well as overcrowding, sometimes three or four to a bed, there were filthy, stinking sanitary conditions. Decomposing corpses were unmoved until claimed by relatives or Poor Law officials. There were commissions of investigation, but little was done.

In May 1750, at The Old Bailey in London, prisoners "accompanied by the most putrid vapors most subtle and volatile" awaited their turn in court. The room was hot, close, and crowded. Four of the six judges on the bench died within ten days, including the Lord Mayor of London. Sir John Pringle, physician and medical historian, wrote, *Two or three counsel, one of the under sheriffs, several of the jury and others present to the amount of forty died; without making allowances for those of lower rank, and without including any of those who did not die within a fortnight.* Judges at the Bailey carry a nosegay of flowers to this day.

More people in the 18th century died of jail fever than were executed.

In 1750, Dr. James Lind of the British Navy blamed the spread of ship fever on dirty clothing and hammocks. He fumigated them and insisted on other standards of hygiene without knowing that lice and their feces, hidden in the clothes and bedding, transmitted the infection. This pragmatic approach saved many lives and gave the British Navy a tactical advantage over the French and Spanish with whom they were at war. Dr. James Lind is also known for showing that scurvy—a common affliction of sailors— was due to the absence of fresh fruit in the diet, eventually leading to the discovery of vitamin C.

Napoleon's Grande Armée famously retreated from Moscow in 1812. Of his six hundred thousand men, only thirty thousand made it back to France. They were lousy. Typhus had started to afflict them on the way into Russia. Starvation, the Tsar's guerilla army, and typhus killed them on the way out.

Typhus appears in 19th-century literature. Leo Tolstoy, Anton Chekhov, Charles Dickens, and Charlotte Brontë all refer to its lethal qualities. "What fast friends," says Dickens, "picturesqueness and typhus often are." Dr. Anton Chekhov wrote a short story in the voice of a man with delirium entitled "Typhus."

In 1906, Howard Taylor Ricketts, a physician scientist from Ohio, showed that Rocky Mountain spotted fever was transmitted by a tick. Three years later, he showed that *tabardillo*, a typhus-like illness scourging Mexico City, was transmitted by the body louse. *Tabardo* means "red cloak"—a reference to the rash. Ricketts caught the disease and died at the age of thirty-nine. At about the same time, the French bacteriologist Charles Nicolle showed that lice, in particular lice feces, transmitted typhus.

A decade passed. In 1916, Stanislaus von Prowazek, a Czech micro-biologist, and the Brazilian Henrique da Rocha Lima were working in Germany because they had been trapped there by the war. In a hospital filled with typhus patients, they discovered, at last, the bacterium that causes the disease. It was a small, stumpy, rod-shaped bacterium tinting pink on the Gram stain just like *Yersinia pestis*. Both investigators caught typhus. Prowazek died. Rocha Lima recovered, and he named the bacteria *Rickettsia prowazeki* in honor of his deceased comrade in science.

Typhus was resurgent in the First World War. A quarter of a million people died in Serbia alone, including 25 percent of the doctors, from this disease. A *rickettsial* bacteria caused a less severe form of typhus also trans-mitted by lice—it became known as trench fever.

Typhus surged again with the Second World War. Eastern Europe bore the brunt. This pandemic did not occur in isolation. Scarlet fever, diphtheria, dysentery, and tuberculosis were its companions.

Thirty recognized species of *rickettsia* cause disease in humans. They are transmitted by mosquito, flea, chigger, tick, or louse. Rocky Mountain spot-ted fever, ehrlichiosis, anaplasmosis, tsutsugamushi fever, and Mediterranean fever (fièvre boutonneuse) are the names of some of them. Many animals are scourged by *rickettsiae* that do not cause disease in humans.

Each year in the US, about five people die from typhus. The cases are sporadic across the country and they happen during the coldest months of the year. Typhus is caught from the flying squirrel, *Glaucomys volans*, which is a known host of *R prowazeki* and nests in the attics of houses during the winter. Flying squirrel typhus is also seen in the cold mountainous regions of Africa and South America. The exact means of transmission is unknown. Lice are not involved.

In 1970, Lynn Margulis published *Origin of Eukaryotic Cells*. *Eukary-otic* means cells that have a nucleus surrounded by a membrane and spe-cialized little organs, or organelles. These are the types of cell that make up our bodies. One of the organelles is the mitochondrion. The idea, first proposed by Konstantin Mereschowski in 1905 and quickly forgotten, is that mitochondria are bacteria that live symbiotically in our eukaryotic cells, and because they are contributing energy, it is a selective advantage not to fight their presence.

Mitochondria are symbiotic bacteria, as are *chloroplasts* in plants. They have their own DNA, which may be damaged by antibiotics. To this day, antibodies cannot decide if mitochondria are self or other. A liver disease called primary biliary cholangitis is caused by the immune system attacking mitochondria, not recognizing them as "self." Anti-mitochondrial antibodies can be detected and are diagnostic of the disease. With evolution over time, mitochondria have given 90 percent of their genes away. The three hundred genes that remain concentrate on the manufacture and storage of energy.

Sperm have mitochondria. They need the energy mitochondria generate to make their long journey to the ovary. When they merge with the ovary to form the *zygote*, the sperm's mitochondria are not incorporated. So, all the mitochondria in your body come from your mother.

What is most surprising about the mitochondria, those powerhouses of the body, is that they most resemble a *rickettsial* organism. And the *rickettsial* organism they most resemble is *Rickettsia prowazeki*.

The last recorded outbreak of epidemic typhus was in 1997, in Burundi. Over 45,000 people in refugee camps suffered from infection. The mortality was low by previous standards because they were given chloramphenicol or tetracycline, antibiotics that first came into use in the 1950s.

In 2012, I went out with my family for a picnic on the banks of the Hudson River. The Walkway Over the Hudson bridge stood in the distance. My sons, then aged ten and eight, were both bitten by ticks, as they had been running through the long grass at the edges of the woods. My wife and I were not bitten. We carefully removed ticks from the boys. Fortunately, they were large ticks, or wood ticks. The ones that transmit infections are deer ticks and they are tiny and difficult to see.

Four days later, as I walked up the stairs of the hospital, I felt, in midstep, as if the world and I had abruptly changed. I was freezing cold and shivering. Shaking, I walked into the Intensive Care Unit, sat on a chair, and said, "[Expletive deleted], I feel cold." A blanket was put around my shoulders, and my temperature was taken. It was 104.5 degrees Fahrenheit, and I was then put in a wheelchair and taken to the Emergency Room. It didn't take them long to diagnose me. My white cell count was low. My platelets were 40,000, also low. My liver function tests were slightly abnormal. My friend Amy, the Emergency Room doctor, told me I had a fine rash over my shoulders.

"You mean I've got typhus?"

"No, mate." She was Australian. "*Anaplasmosis.* The typhus of the Mid-Hudson Valley. Still, they are both *rickettsial* organisms, aren't they? Are you allergic to tetracycline?"

"No . . . I . . . no."

"Good. We'll get you started on some IV."

It began to sink in.

I wasn't going to make it to poker tonight.

I could see intensely colored patterns forming on the white ceiling above me, which is not uncommon with temperatures of 105 degrees Fahrenheit. I didn't mind. I actually enjoyed the light show. At the same time, my mind was racing. Over 150 million years ago, *rickettsial* organisms evolved. You can bet that as soon as my, our, ancestors came along, they were infected by them. These pathogens are heirlooms. They lived in biting insects. Untold millions of people have died from *rickettsial* infections and I've got one right now. *Rickettsia* are roaming though my blood, but I'm going to be okay because of Louis Pasteur, Howard Ricketts, Stanislaus Prowazek, Henrique Rocha Lima, Alexander Fleming, Howard Florey, Ernst Chain, and Yellapragada Subbarow (under whose supervision the first tetracycline antibiotic was discovered by Benjamin Duggar).

The nurse was putting up the IV. *Good work, Amy.* Her name was Amy, too. The needle went straight in the first time. Patterns, ceiling. I started laughing.

"What is it, Doc?"

"These *rickettsiae* I have in my blood could not be subdued without my immune system, which couldn't work without the *rickettsiae* living in each of my cells. I wouldn't be here—none of us would—without the *rickettsiae* in our cells called mitochondria. It's a reunion, a party! Every cell in my body is driven by mitochondria. Do they recognize one another? Distant cousins?"

I heard Amy the nurse talking to Amy the doctor. "He is clearly delirious."

CHAPTER 6

COUGHING BLOOD: TUBERCULOSIS

N oel Browne, Irish physician and later Minister of Health, was born near Athlone in the center of Ireland. The following is from his autobiography, *Against the Tide*. The year is 1922. He is eight years old.

An expression of total desolation on both my parents' faces as we met them at the station made it clear to all of us that something dreadful had happened. A Dublin medical specialist had confirmed that our father suffered from severe pulmonary tuberculosis. Although they did not know it at the time my mother was also infected with the same disease. They in turn could have infected their children. I recall an infant sister Annie, leaving our house in a tiny white coffin. She had died of miliary tuberculosis. My elder brother Jody had, along with an untreated hare lip, a grossly deformed hunchback spine from tuberculosis. Although intelligent he could never attend school.

In addition to Jody and the infant who died, my mother, myself, and two sisters became infected with tuberculosis, and with the exception of myself, all have since died from the disease.

Jody, the brother with the hunchback, had Pott's disease, a tuberculous bone infection of the spine. A seven-thousand-year-old etching of Pott's is found on the wall of an Egyptian tomb.

The first written description of tuberculosis comes to us from 300 BCE in *Huangdi Neijing*, a Chinese medical text. The word used for the disease is Ao (癆), meaning *consumption*.

> *Persistent cough, wasting, coughing of blood, fever, shortness of breath.*
> *After months or years of suffering it brings death to the sufferer.*
> *Afterwards it is transferred to others until the whole family is wiped out.*

This text precisely describes the fate of Noel Browne's family—two thousand years before it happened and from three thousand miles away. And the word *consumption* and its context are the same in Chinese and English.

The consensus is that the bacteria *Mycobacterium tuberculosis* (*MTb*) arose in what is now Somalia, the Horn of Africa, twenty thousand years ago. The oldest proven examples of our ongoing human tuberculosis pandemic, dating from nine thousand years ago, are the skeletal remains of a mother in her twenties holding a child. The bones were found in a village now submerged in the Mediterranean off the coast of Atlit Yam, Israel. *MTb* DNA was isolated from these remains.

Reference to consumption, as a divine threat, is found in the Bible:

> *The LORD shall smite thee with a consumption, and with fever, and*
> *with an inflammation, and with an extreme burning, and with the*
> *sword, and with blasting, and with mildew; and they shall pursue thee*
> *until thou perish.*

~Deuteronomy 28:22 (King James Bible)

This passage is also in the Torah, concerning the time the Israelites were in Egypt, and uses the word *Schachepheth*, which meant "wasting disease." The modern Hebrew word for tuberculosis is *Schachefet*.

The ancient cultures of Egypt, Persia, Greece, Rome, and China all knew and wrote of consumption. *MTb* DNA was extracted from Egyptian mummies in the 1990s—the first use of such technology. Tuberculosis did not flourish at a pandemic level until the cold, crowded medieval cities of Europe dominated the continent. It spread from those cities to everywhere in the world that had not yet seen the disease.

What are these bacteria that have tormented us for at least nine thousand years? Of the 190 species of mycobacteria so far discovered, nine cause tuberculosis in humans. About sixty others can cause different types of disease depending on the state of your immunity. The oldest, *M ulcerans,* originated 150 million years ago in Africa and is found in slow-flowing water in many parts of the world. In humans it causes chronic indolent ulcers on the shins. Mycobacteria have thick waxy membranes, which make them difficult to treat, and they divide slowly, some taking twenty days.

Leprosy is caused by a mycobacteria and it was the first of the species to be discovered by the Norwegian Gerhard Hansen in 1873. To this day, leprosy is called Hansen's disease. In 2008, 135 years later, a second mycobacteria was discovered that causes the same, or a very similar, disease, usually in people of Mexican or Caribbean origin. Hansen's bacteria is called *Mycobacterium leprae*; the second is known as *Mycobacterium lepromatis.* These two bacteria diverged into distinct species ten million years ago. There are more species of mycobacteria in sub-Saharan Africa than anywhere else in the world, which is an indicator of their place of origin.

MAN BITES COW

From amebae to goldfish, from elephants to parrots to man, many animals are infected with mycobacteria. *Mycobacterium bovis* infects cows. It was thought that man must have come in contact with the disease when we domesticated cattle 12,000 years ago. However, human tuberculosis and cow tuberculosis diverged, which is to say they developed different DNA making them separate organisms 113,000 years ago. So, *we* infected cattle and many other animals besides. Once humans have infected cows, cows can in turn infect other humans—which is why you shouldn't drink unpasteurized milk.

When mummies with Pott's disease who had died at various times between 700 and 1200 were found in the Atacama Desert of Peru, it threw another widely held belief into question. Surely tuberculosis was brought to the Americas by the Spanish conquistadores and other European colonizers? Well, it was, no doubt. But before then it was brought by seals from Africa.

When the mycobacteria were extracted from the Peruvian mummies' spines, it showed the DNA of *Mycobacterium pinnepedi*, the bacteria that causes disease in sea lions and seals. *Pinnepedi* means "fin feet." However, northern hemisphere seals are not infected. Man infected seals in Africa. Over the course of many generations, the infection was passed from seal to seal along the coast of Antarctica from the Cape of Good Hope to Cape Horn. Peruvian seal hunters acquired the infection from hunting, killing, and eating these animals, and when infected, passed it on to other humans. In line with this is the outbreak in 2008 of *M pinnepedi* tuberculosis in sea lions in a Netherlands zoo. Six of twenty-five zoo workers were infected. Tuberculosis infection is an occupational hazard of zoo workers. Another characteristic of mycobacteria is that they jump species unpredictably. There are documented records of bidirectional transmission of bacteria causing tuberculosis between humans and camels, humans and elephants, humans and goats, and humans and parrots.

Tuberculosis is highly contagious. As few as eight bacteria breathed in from recently coughed-into air may cause tuberculosis. As we have seen, it is predominantly a pulmonary disease, at least in people of European origin, yet it may affect any tissue in the body. In the disease scrofula, tuberculous swelling of lymph nodes in the neck and elsewhere may be thought of as buboes in slow motion. Over several years, they break down and discharge pus. They are not hot and inflamed; they are cold abscesses. Patients with scrofula present an awful sight. This disease was recognized in Europe in the 8th, 9th, and 10th centuries. It was called the King's Evil and could be cured if the king touched you. Phillip of France used *le toucher Royale*, and Edward the Confessor would do the same in England. This ability to cure was evidence of the ruler's divine appointment to the throne.

Shakespeare writes in *Macbeth*:

> *Strangely visited people,*
> *All swoln and ulcerous, pitiful to the eye,*
> *The mere despair of surgery, he cures;*
> *Hanging a golden stamp around their necks,*
> *Put on with holy prayers; and 'tis spoken,*

To the succeeding royalty he leaves
The healing benediction.

The practice of the Royal Touch continued until Louis XV in France and George I in England put a stop to it. Voltaire said he had lost faith in the therapy when one of Louis XIV's mistresses died of scrofula in spite of the king's touch.

The plague of tuberculosis expanded as never before in the cities and megalopolises of the 18th, 19th, and 20th centuries. It was abetted by overcrowding, poverty, ignorance, poor working conditions, poor ventilation, primitive sanitation, smog, and malnutrition—but these factors were rarely understood or acknowledged.

In *The Life and Death of Mr. Badman*, a moralistic tract written by John Bunyan in 1680, he describes his character's demise:

> *I cannot so properly say that he died of one disease, for there were many that had consented, and laid their heads together to bring him to his end. He was dropsical, he was Consumptive, he was surfeited, he was gouty, and, as some say he had the tang of pox in his bowels. Yet the captain of all these men of death that came against him to take him away, was the Consumption, for it was that, that brought him down to the grave.*

Bunyan makes a point. Mr. Badman has other diseases, or "co-morbidities" in contemporary medical jargon, which render Mr. Badman more likely to reactivate his consumption. The disease has gone by many names: Phthisis, King's Evil, Graveyard Cough, Robber of Youth, White Plague, Asthenia, aesthenia, acid-fast infection (after 1882), tuberculosis—or, as Bunyan aptly called it, "the captain of all these men of death."

CONSUMED BY PASSION

Tuberculosis is merciless. It progresses slowly and unrelentingly. You cough, you cough blood, you waste away, and you are ultimately consumed.

Consumption made its way into many homes. The literary Brontë sisters' mother, Maria (née Bramwell), died at thirty-nine from an unknown disease after having delivered six children, five girls and a boy. The Brontës lived in the Haworth Parsonage, Yorkshire, England, in a large, well-aired house. Two of the girls, Elizabeth and Maria, died at nine and ten years of age respectively. Between the years 1848 and 1849, Anne (*Agnes Grey*) at twenty-nine, Emily (*Wuthering Heights*) at thirty, and Branwell at thirty-one, all died of consumption. Charlotte (*Jane Eyre*), the oldest, died at forty in 1855. Their father, Patrick, the parson, returned to Ireland, the country of his birth, for the last few years of his eighty-four-year life span. From the impact on the Brontë family, it is easy to understand how consumption could be portrayed as a genetic disease. Entire families were wiped out, and the number of unknown families afflicted in a similar way to the Brontës would have been boundless.

In England as a whole, in the cities in particular, and in London most of all, tuberculosis was increasing in incidence by the beginning of the 19th century. In the capital, one in four deaths were caused by the disease. Understanding its cause and determining effective treatment were no closer than they had been two hundred years earlier. It would be understandable to say a thousand years earlier, but in 1882 accurate descriptions of the pathology of consumption had been made and René Laennec had invented the stethoscope (1816), enabling the physician to hear the physical signs of tuberculosis affecting the lungs.

The prevalence of consumption as a lethal disease that was also part of everyday life led some to romanticize it. When Charlotte Brontë said of her sister Anne, who was dying at age twenty-nine, "Consumption, I am aware, is a flattering malady," it jars, until you understand that this attitude was the norm in her social class. Refined suffering with superior spirituality and intelligence was the key to beauty. Passion was everything. Consumptive allure with much swooning helped women distance themselves from the squalor of the 19th century. It was thought that consumption required a special soul to acquire it. Women were thin, coughing blood delicately into lace handkerchiefs. Transparency and whiteness of the skin, a flushed cheek, and red full lips from fever were the look of the age. It became fashionable for healthy women to starve themselves and apply artificial whiteners to the skin. In Paris, there was a similar attitude. Alexandre Dumas said, "It was good form to cough blood with the least emotion and to die before thirty." A society doctor of the time told a patient on her first visit, "You feel well, you eat well, you sleep well. Follow my instructions and I will soon remove every appearance of health, I assure you."

There were many explanations for consumption. The aforementioned Laennec strongly believed it was caused by melancholia or occasionally excessive joy. Lack of exercise, particularly among married women, was proposed as a cause, as was too much dancing, especially the waltz.

For a hundred years, romantic ideas, where passion is placed above reason, held sway. "Do you not see," said one poet, "how necessary a world of pains and troubles is to school an Intelligence and make it a soul?"

The poet was John Keats.

He had graduated as an apothecary at Guy's Hospital and wrote from his experiences on the ward:

> *The weariness, the fever, and the fret*
> *Here, where men sit and hear each other groan;*
> *Where palsy shakes a few, sad, last grey hairs*
> *Where youth grows pale and spectre-thin and dies;*
> *Where but to think is to be full of sorrow*
> *And leaden-eyed despairs.*

~"Ode to a Nightingale," 1819

Keats's death in Rome—where he had gone to seek a more forgiving climate in a house by the Spanish Steps—has been much described. He is winnowed to the core. The extent to which it is romantic may be judged by the descriptions of his friend and companion to the end, Joseph Severn. He describes Keats crying for opiates, waking in the night and weeping that he was still alive. He writes:

> *He is now in a most deplorable state. His stomach is ruined and the state*
> *of his mind is the worst possible for one in his condition . . . It is most*
> *distressing to see a mind like his in the deplorable state in which it is . . . I*
> *fear the prospect is hopeless.*

Tact restrained him from mentioning the *fetor ex oris*, the foul breath of the consumptive.

Keats himself had written: *Now more than ever it seems rich to die, to cease upon the midnight hour with no pain*, thus outlining the aim of palliative care to come.

The poet Percy Bysshe Shelley, another consumptive, wrote:

> *Peace, peace! He is not dead, he doth not sleep*
> *He hath awakened from the dream of life.*

There is nothing romantic whatsoever about dying at twenty-five years of age from a progressive disease that wastes you away, causes a characteristic unpleasant halitosis, and leads to a persistent hacking cough so violent that you lose control of your bladder, that produces green sputum and amounts of blood that may cause you to drown in your own secretions, and that literally consumes you. And yet, literature is filled with paeans to consumption.

"He died of his unrequited love for Fanny Brawne."

" . . . of his sensitive poetic soul."

" . . . of an unfavorable critique in the *Quarterly Review*."

"Consumption confers beauty on the sufferer."

"It requires a special soul to die from it."

Keats died from infection with *Mycobacterium tuberculosis*, a bacteria acquired from nursing his brother who died himself of the disease at the age of eighteen.

It's not difficult to understand romanticizing death at a young age. Suffering is better if it has a redemptive quality. The cult of sensibility acts to console, to make the death of a loved one more bearable. How else to palliate the mind over large numbers of young people dealing with slow, premature, and inescapable death? Yet as the century wore on and evidence of a contagious explanation began to appear more likely, the cult of romanticism began to fade. The artist Amedeo Modigliani died of tuberculosis in 1920, but by then it was completely unfashionable.

In Yorkshire, just down the road from the Brontës, the town of Haworth was hell. The workers were poor and lived in overcrowded slums with contaminated water. Forty percent of children died before the age of six and overall life expectancy was twenty-five years. There was little talk of souls and the elegance of the consumptive.

Physicians had various explanations for the disease. In America, William Osler at Johns Hopkins Hospital in Baltimore remarked with insight, "Tuberculosis is a social disease with some medical aspects."

Often, they blamed the patient.

In a textbook of medicine from 1881, the year before the bacteria was discovered, you may read the following on the *aetiology* (cause) of tuberculosis:

The disease is a hereditary weakness, insomuch as whole families have made their exits through consumption. The Irish are particularly prone.

It is due to the inheritance of a flawed, usually weak and delicate constitution. This is the tubercular diathesis.

Profound emotions are to be avoided particularly in young women who are exceptionally vulnerable.

The poor are more likely to acquire the infection because of their predilection for unsound habits.

Habits of life are of the greatest importance. Self-abuse, intemperance and sexual misbehavior predispose to tuberculosis. The disease is a consequence of these personal defects.

In contrast, the physician/poet Thomas Beddoes wrote,

The disorder shows itself in a different form in poor families, where children are fed on water-gruel and potatoes. The countenance is then pale, bloated, and what medical writers term cachectic. The upper lip is particularly tumid. The eyes are dull instead of bright. Privation and pain necessarily produce ill temper and stupidity.

And philosopher Friedrich Engels wrote,

The bad air of London is the highest degree favorable to the development of Consumption. Pale, lank, narrow chested, hollow eyed, ghosts whom

one passes at every step. These languid flabby faces are incapable of the
slightest energetic expression.

Many events of the era have been romanticized: *La Bohème, La Dame*
aux Camelias, the deaths of Chopin at thirty-seven (though he coughed
with infinite grace), Chekhov at forty-four, and Robert Louis Stevenson
in the South Pacific at age forty-four. As poignant as those events were,
the most romantic, and world-changing, event of the era was when Robert
Koch revolutionized medicine from a corner of his apartment in Germany
in 1882. He identified *Mycobacterium tuberculosis*, a bacteria, as the cause of
consumption. Someone should write an opera about it.

CONSUMPTION
BECOMES TUBERCULOSIS

Tuberculosis started to infect *Homo sapiens* in the Horn of Africa about
twenty thousand years ago and we carried it around the world. The disease
is ancient in the Indian subcontinent, in Europe, in China, and Japan. It
continued at a low level until the great cities of the world became breeding
grounds for the disease. Some tuberculosis reached South America, carried
by seals infected in South Africa. European colonizers took the disease to
populations in North America, Australia, New Zealand, and the Pacific
islands where the inhabitants represented virgin populations. The indigenous people of these places suffered greatly.

Peaking in Europe in the late 19th century, tuberculosis began to
abate on the back of better social circumstances and possibly improving
immunity.

But even as late as 1939, Noel Browne knew there was no effective
treatment. He wrote, while taking his final exams in medicine:

I was sleepy no matter how much I rested and I was losing weight. Chest
X-rays confirmed I had active tuberculosis in both lungs.
A woman who acted as domestic help declined to come into my room.
Overnight I had joined the ghetto of the tuberculosis lepers in Irish life. I

told my fiancé that for her own protection she should forget our friendship;
remarkably and happily for me, this she did not do.

A nearly hysterical fear of tuberculosis was universal. It affected
all classes as there was no certain cure. With the best possible intentions
I was subjected to many extraordinary drugs, some of them positively
dangerous, and all useless. Sanocycin, a gold preparation, caused a blood
disorder and I became very ill. All else having failed it was decided in
1942 to operate on my lungs.

In 1948, aged thirty-five years, Noel Browne had not died. He was
elected to the Parliament of Ireland, the Dáil Éireann, and was made Minister of Health.

As a doctor I was especially unhappy about general medical needs and
the virtually nonexistent tuberculosis programme and this powerfully
motivated me to make progress in our hospitals and especially to curb
tuberculosis. A clear plan of action was quickly outlined. First, limitation
of the disease by isolation of sources of infection. Next, freely available
X ray services and a BCG innoculation service [BCG stands for Bacille
Calmette Guerin, a vaccine against tuberculosis]. We launched a new
"clean food" code backed with a press, radio and film campaign directed to
educate the public in methods of hygienic food preparation, sale and usage.
We set up the National Blood Transfusion Organization.

Fresh air was considered important. Patients in sanatoria were encouraged to stick their heads out of the window. Two pints of Guinness were
to be taken daily as part of the regime, not necessarily with the head out
of the window.

A year after these measures were established, streptomycin—an antibiotic that cures tuberculosis—became available in Ireland. The longed-
for miracle was effective at first, but gradually it stopped working as the
bacteria became resistant. It was not long before other drugs—isoniazid,
ethambutol, pyrazinamide—were also found to be effective, so the problem
of resistance was overcome with the use of a three-drug regimen. This led
to a convincing cure for the disease, at least for the next fifty years. The

incidence of tuberculosis began to slowly decline in Ireland in the 1950s, and by the 1970s it had all but disappeared.

Just as St. Patrick had cast the snakes out of Ireland, Noel Browne cast out the tubercule bacillus. He took streptomycin himself, which left him deaf in one ear, a well-recognized side effect. He retired with his wife to County Galway where he died aged eighty-one years.

With the advent of anti-tuberculous antibiotics in the 1950s, the disease was controlled in the developed world. The BCG vaccine referred to above leaves public health services advisors divided. It is given to about a hundred million children yearly, particularly in Asia.

Despite knowledge of the bacteria that causes the disease and effective antibiotic treatment, there are currently more people infected with tuberculosis than ever.

We have a relationship with this bacterium. It may infect us and lie dormant in immune cells called *macrophages* that gather together and imprison the microbe. It is alive but not replicating as it lies there in a swelling called a granuloma or a tubercule. One-third of today's humans are infected with *Mycobacterium tuberculosis* in this latent state. One in three, that's 1.8 billion of the world's population. In the cities of the world in the 19th century, the infection rate was more like nine out of ten. So, are we winning this struggle with tuberculosis?

We are immune but just barely. If you impair immunity to any degree—if you take hydrochloric acid–lowering medicines for indigestion, if you take steroids for any reason, if you are getting older, if you are malnourished, if you have other diseases such as diabetes, chronic obstructive pulmonary disease, chronic leukemia, or suffer from renal failure—you run the risk that your latent tuberculosis will reactivate. Between 5 and 20 percent of people with latent tuberculosis reactivate their disease. The risk in people with AIDS is much higher. In most HIV patients with latent tuberculosis, it is reactivated as their immunity becomes compromised. HIV-positive people are routinely tested for tuberculosis and vice versa. One in four AIDS deaths is caused by tuberculosis.

While most of those infected with *Mycobacterium tuberculosis* have a latent infection, ten million people have active tuberculosis, and of those, 1.6 million died in 2018. It is the leading infectious cause of death in the world. Tuberculosis is particularly prevalent in sub-Saharan Africa. Over the last twenty years, it has been on the rise for two primary reasons.

The first is the association with AIDS. In 2019, forty million people were infected with HIV worldwide.

The second is drug resistance. Cases of drug-resistant tuberculosis have been reported in most countries of the world, including Europe and North America. The highest incidence is in Russia and countries of the former USSR. There is multi-drug resistant tuberculosis, *MDR*, and extensively drug resistant tuberculosis, *XDR*.

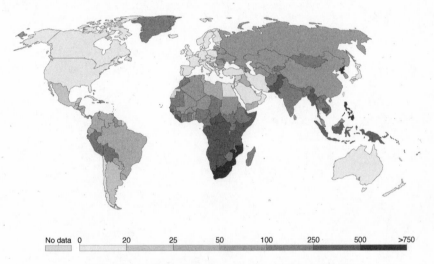

Distribution of tuberculosis in the world as of 2016 (cases per 100,000 people). Our World in Data, https://ourworldindata.org/grapher/incidence-of-tuberculosis-sdgs, CC BY 3.0.

To date, there are suitable antibiotic alternatives for the treatment of patients suffering from these forms of the disease, but they are inferior to first-line drugs. Treatment options are shrinking as the disease is expanding.

The human plague that started at least nine thousand years ago shows no sign of abating.

CHAPTER 7

. . . .

THE GREAT
IMITATOR: SYPHILIS

A s humans came to live in the ever-enlarging cities of Europe from the 14th century on, a steep price in suffering was paid in the painful mortality of infectious diseases. Forty percent of children born died before age five from measles, diphtheria, and smallpox, to name only three. Adults lived at constant risk of death from plague, typhus, tuberculosis, and typhoid. Then, at the beginning of the 16th century, there emerged another, slower malady. It is mentioned obliquely, with euphemism, under one's breath, because . . . it is transmitted by sex.

Girolamo Fracastoro, born in 1472 in Verona, then part of the Republic of Venice, was appointed professor of the university at age nineteen. Copernicus was his contemporary. He invented the word *fomites*, meaning the contaminated effluents of a patient (see Chapter 4). He is famous in the history of medicine for three additional achievements—for proposing in 1546 that epidemic diseases are transmitted by tiny particles or spores, for giving a concise and accurate clinical account of pulmonary tuberculosis, and for inventing the word *syphilis*. He had written a poem about a shepherd who displeased Apollo and was punished with a disfiguring disease. The shepherd's name was Syphilis. It sounded more refined than the "pox" or "morbus gallicus" ("the French disease"), which were other labels commonly used. Fracastoro treated syphilis, epidemic in the city from about 1530 on, and became rich doing so. Titian painted his portrait in exchange for therapy. A crater on the moon is named after him. That's quite a career.

The contemporary diarist Marino Sanudo had no doubt that Columbus's men brought syphilis back to Spain from the "new" world—a matter that's been debated for 520 years. The weight of evidence suggests Sanudo was right. After all, the very first known outbreak of syphilis was in Barcelona in 1494 after which its spread was abetted by war. The French invaded Italy using Spanish mercenaries, some of whom had sailed with Columbus. They marched into Milan in 1496 trailed by camp followers. Victory was easy at first, although the war was to last for thirty years. Milan promptly experienced an outbreak of the "French" disease. As Sanudo wrote, *Heavenly influences, and the arrival of the French in Italy have brought a new infirmity. It originates from the private parts and is spread by intercourse and no other means. There is fever, pains in the joints and a blistering rash.*

The speed with which syphilis spread was astounding. By 1497, it was in Aberdeen, a thriving Scottish seaport. There they called it "gore" or "grandgore." In the following year in Edinburgh, "light women" were sent to the island of Inchkeith on pain of branding on the face as the disease in "Auld Reekie" (Edinburgh) was obviously their fault.

Syphilis seemed to be everywhere in Europe at once. The entire world was the next logical step, and the malady obliged. Vasco da Gama rounded the Cape in 1497, and in 1498 syphilis is recorded in Bombay (Mumbai). In 1505, it is reported in Guangzhou, and by 1526 it is in the cities of Japan.

This early version of syphilis was more virulent than that described today because the world was a virgin population and had no natural immunity. During that period of exploration and colonization, the indigenous peoples of the Americas got smallpox, measles, influenza, yellow fever, and tuberculosis from Europe. The Spanish got syphilis and helped to distribute it worldwide.

A hundred years later, Voltaire wrote, *On their flippant way through Italy, the French army carelessly picked up Genoa, Naples, and syphilis. They lost Genoa and Naples, but . . .*

It starts with a painless genital ulcer. Personal accounts of this odd but unmistakable blemish are hard to find outside of medical literature.

The word is chancre, similar to cancer, but it is not a cancer. It may not be noticeable at first, especially in women. The local lymph nodes swell. They, too, are painless. Some will have ulcers on the mouth, the finger, or the rectum. Those afflicted may feel ill as if with influenza. It comes on from three to ninety days after sexual intercourse with infected persons, usually within twenty-eight days. It lasts a week or so, and then it goes away. Syphilis is a stroll along the Grand Canal compared to the plague.

It returns.

Syphilis is caused by the spirochete bacterium *Treponema pallidum*. Although the disease was quickly determined to be sexually transmitted, it would be five hundred years before the proximate cause was discovered and a further fifty before penicillin, the absolute cure, was in use. The organism and the immune system struggle at a complex chemical level. The chancre is the consequence of this struggle. And then it heals up without a scar! Victory to the immune system!

This pale, simple bacterium returns for a second time.

The first protospirochete from which all spirochetes on Earth are descended arose three billion years ago. A multitude of bacteria from seven genera are found in the mouths and intestines of many animals, including humans, but they are inert and do not cause disease. Or very few cause disease. *Treponema pallidum ssp pallidum* causes syphilis, *Treponema pallidum ssp pretenue* causes yaws, and *Borrelia burgdorferi* causes Lyme disease. Some spirochetes in our mouths cooperate with other organisms to cause gingivitis.

They divide every thirty-three hours, which is slow by bacterial standards (by comparison, *E. coli* divides every twenty minutes). Sometimes the treponemes reside in humans in a latent state, replicating as infrequently as once every six months. So, after the chancre goes away, a few bacilli remain, doubling unhurriedly.

SECONDARY SYPHILIS

In 1500, Benvenuto Cellini was born in Florence. He became a master goldsmith, sculptor, soldier, musician, and artist. It is the Renaissance, after all. Before he died, seventy-one years later, he wrote an autobiography in which he describes what it is like to have secondary syphilis.

> It was true indeed that I got the sickness; I believe I caught it from that fine young servant-girl whom I was keeping . . .
>
> The French disease, for it was that, remained in me for more than four months dormant before it showed itself and then it broke out over my whole body in one instant. It was not like what one commonly observes, but covered my flesh with blisters the size of a sixpence and rose colored. The doctors could not call it the French disease although I told them why I thought it was that. I went on treating myself in accordance with their methods, but derived no benefit. At last, then, I resolved on taking the Wood against the advice of my first physicians in Rome and I took it with the most scrupulous discipline and rules of abstinence that could be thought of, and after a few days I perceived in me a great amendment. The result was that in fifty days I was cured and sound as a cockroach.

By "taking the wood," Cellini means oil of the guaiac tree, also known as holy wood or *Lignam Vitae*, the wood of life. From the 15th to the 20th centuries, there were three specific treatments for syphilis: holy wood, the salts of mercury, and hot baths.

Benvenuto's description and self-diagnosis are impressive. This is secondary syphilis. He felt ill with his rash, was nauseous, lost weight, had an intermittent sore throat with ulcers in his mouth, aches and pains, swollen lymph nodes, and hair coming out of his head in clumps. He went from looking moth eaten to bald. He catalogs his experience: *It's been a week now that I have felt fine. Except I'm bald. I'm not quite so relieved as I was when the chancre went away and I have taken the treatment. So far, touch Wood, va bene.*

The disease returns.

How do the spirochetes persist? Do they hide in sanctuary somewhere in the body where immunity does not impact them? Are there such sites? We don't know, even today. They survive somehow, then reactivate to kill the host. Ultimately, they are victorious. Victory at what cost? Death of the host means death of the spirochete. Unless it has been passed on to another. Only in this way does *Treponema pallidum* live on in the world.

If Columbus and his men brought syphilis back from Hispaniola to Spain, it begs the question: How did it get to Hispaniola? In the rain forests of Africa, gorillas, chimpanzees, baboons, and smaller primates are infected with a disease called yaws. Humans also suffer from yaws. It is caused by a spirochete very similar to *Treponema pallidum*. Yaws is not transmitted from mother to fetus. It is transmitted from mother to child and from child to child through nonsexual contact. It is mostly found in tropical zones where there is poverty, physical closeness, and relatively poor hygiene. Where the road ends, yaws begins.

Yaws usually starts on the lower limbs with a painless red swelling and an innocuous enlargement of the local lymph nodes. This sore is the mother yaw. It lasts weeks or months and then disappears. *Treponemes* disseminate in the secondary stage and cause multiple skin lesions called daughter yaws. They are small and painful, often involving an inflammation of the bone's lining, which is called *periostitis*. These lesions also heal.

Ten percent of untreated victims develop deforming tertiary yaws resulting in sabre-shaped tibias and other skeletal deformities. A distant similarity to the stages of syphilis can be noted, but unlike syphilis, yaws rarely crosses the placenta, seldom attacks the central nervous system, and does not affect the heart. *Homo erectus* was a human primate that lived for 1.5 million years, which is far longer than we, *Homo sapiens*, have been here. They became extinct 250,000 years ago. Bony lesions on skeletal remains shows they suffered from yaws. So, yaws is an heirloom infection that was waiting for us when we first appeared on Earth.

In the 1950s, the WHO almost eradicated yaws by mass treating of susceptible populations with the antibiotic erythromycin. The key word is *almost*. There was an incidence reduction of 95 percent. Regrettably, with the ponies of the apocalypse in Africa, it has returned to its previous levels, which is from 1 to 20 percent of the population, depending on the environment.

DNA studies show there is 99.63 percent similarity in the 1,200,000 genetic base pairs that make up the yaws and syphilis spirochetes.

LATENT SYPHILIS

In June 1606, William Shakespeare wakes one morning in his lodgings in St Olave's parish, London. He is forty-two years old. He has syphilis, or what he would call "the pocks," although "the gore" was used nearly as often. He is sensitive about his baldness. Both syphilis and smallpox cause baldness, accounting for the popularity of wigs.

What's more, there are rumors of plague. When are there not? If forty or more deaths are reported in a day, the playhouses will be closed.

> *The dead man's knell*
> *Is there scarce asked for who,*
> *And good men's lives*
> *Expire before the flowers in their caps,*
> *Dying or ere they sicken.*

~Macbeth, **Act 4, Scene 3**

Shakespeare walks down Noble Street, across Chepeside, along Watling Street to the drawbridge on the north of the congested bridge. He picks his way through the chickens, pigs, goats, donkeys, and carts. He sees no dogs, as there had been a recent slaughtering of strays. The City Fathers would pay a halfpenny a carcass. If it were to control the plague, so be it. The consequence was more rats.

The smell of excrement is everywhere mingling with the noxious odor of sea coal. It was for this he would take a wherry or a skiff from the city quays to Bankside. Not today. He dwells in London and must be inured to the smell. Each week the city feels more crowded with rustics, immigrants from the countryside desperate to escape the poverty of their life. They come from the length of the land. He pushes past them. He is going for his hot bath on Tooley Street.

At the stone gate, at the southern end of the bridge in the liberties now, a woman approaches. Will sees her clearly. She was in the Tabard that night when he caroused with Ben Johnson—was it a six-month past? He yet recalls her name. Sussex Sarah. At this morning hour, she approaches, a sister of the southbanck, a Winchester goose, drab, whore, punk, beagle.

"Are you a King's man?" She's being sly, drawing a double U, ESS in the air with her finger.

"Get you gone, trull."

"Nay, lion, I am chaste except for sixpence."

Her face is half hidden by a scarf. She has aged ten years in one. He feels anger. In her corrupted body lies the burn, the pocks from France.

Love's fire heats water; Water cools not love.

~Sonnet 154

He masters his repulsion. He glances back at the traitors' heads impaled on poles at the southern end of the bridge. He finds a farthing for her, the smallest glint of love. He has seen the black sore under her cowl, above her right eye. The infinite malady. "Get you back to Lewes. Go this day."

Give them diseases, leaving with thee their lust.
Make use of thy salt hours; season the slaves
For tubs and baths; bring down the rose-cheeked youth to the tub-fast
*   and the diet.*

~Timon of Athens, Act 4, Scene 3

He knocks, enters the bathhouse, and wearily undresses for his treatment in the tub. Each ache, pain, or pang sends an alert. Is this the dreadful end? Like Cesare by our Lady Borgia? Hemings? William by our Lady Herbert?

"Good morrow, Will."

"Good morrow, Phillip. What blessings to cheer the client?"

"You look well, Will. Dost thou eat the blue pill each day?"

"Such salts I take. Until I spit like a bitch. But see my hands."

He holds them out; they tremble forcibly.

"Makes writing elephantine."

"William shakes."

William Shakespeare did not die from syphilis. He died at age fifty-two from an acute febrile illness, possibly typhus. His tremor was a side effect of the mercury salts, treatment for the gore. It may explain why he did not write in the last three years of his life. He had latent disease, between secondary and tertiary syphilis.

TERTIARY SYPHILIS

One in three patients with latent disease develops tertiary syphilis. It returns two to thirty years after secondary syphilis clears up. There are three forms. The first is *gumma*.

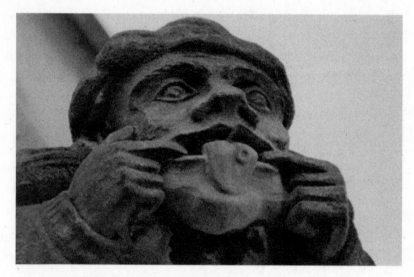

Gargoyle at the Guild Chapel, Stratford-upon-Avon, showing gumma of the tongue. Septemberlegs/Alamy Stock Photo.

These are firm swellings that break out at random in the liver, brain, heart, skin, tongue, bone, and testes and ulcerate in the center. They are painful and particularly malicious when they cause disfiguring ulcers of the face. Secondly, it affects the ascending aorta, causing an aneurysm, a leaking valve, and narrowing of the coronary arteries sufficient to cause a heart attack and sudden death.

It may cause the same painful bone lesions, periostitis, as are seen in yaws. It affects the brain and spinal cord, leading to dementia, epilepsy, and paralysis. There are three primary overlapping forms of late-stage syphilis and the central nervous system: locomotor ataxia, tabes dorsalis, and general paralysis of the insane.

In Paris, 1889, a man stumbles along the sidewalk, lurching into café tables and sending carafes and glasses flying. Waiters run to intervene. He shrugs them off, and, waving his right arm high, he crashes off into the darkness. He appears drunk but is not. He has syphilis of the brain. He cannot maintain his balance. He has locomotor ataxia. It is known to this day as Maupassant's sign.

Guy de Maupassant came to Paris from Normandy at the age of twenty. His civil service job was boring. The delights of the capital, on the other hand, were not. On one occasion he astounded his friends by taking six prostitutes one after the other. At twenty-two years of age, he noticed a painless ulcer on his penis. He learned the word chancre.

During *La Belle Époque*, literally "the Beautiful Time" but more often used to mean "the Good Old Days," syphilis was rampant in Paris. As in Elizabethan and Jacobean London and Kinshasa in the 1970s, overcrowding, poverty, and a brisk sex industry were the handmaidens of pestilence. London was the same, in fairness, as were megalopolises around the world.

Paris was the center of that world. A riot of theatre, music halls, banqueting, absinthe, gaiety, Montmartre, *Les Folies Bergère*, and above them all, visible from nearly everywhere, the newly built Eiffel Tower dominating the landscape.

Dr. Alfred Fournier, the eminent Parisian venereologist, estimated that 15 percent of the population was infected with whatever caused syphilis. The doctor then, as now, is the bourgeois keeper of secrets. Only within the brotherhood may he talk of syphilis and its science. In society he will talk discreetly, in euphemisms: lues, specific disease, an inherited neurological disorder, a serious condition, the Neapolitan evil, the great distress, the infinite malady.

When Guy de Maupassant got his diagnosis from Dr. Fournier, he was elated. "I've got the pox!" he shouted. "The real thing! Not the contemptible clap, not the ecclesiastical crystalline, not the bourgeois coxcombs or the leguminous cauliflowers, no-no, the great pox, the one which Francis I died of. The majestic pox, pure and simple; the elegant syphilis."

He saw it as a badge of humanity, of adulthood. Or bravado. Or something. Yet he was going prematurely bald and suffered odd pains, sometimes in his chest. The disease was an open secret whose name must not be spoken.

Guy de Maupassant wrote a story, "Bed 29," in which a hussar, still trim of thigh, learns that his great love Irma is in the hospital. They had been separated by the Franco-Prussian War, in which he had fought and won the Military Cross. She is in the Salpetrière, one of the city's largest hospitals. He is directed to her ward. Above the door is written one word: *Syphilitiques.*

The impact is shocking. All well and good, as this is a medical establishment and the usual taboo does not apply. It is still a slap in the face. Irma is hardly recognizable. She is old, ugly, and ill, her face twisted. She had been raped by Prussians, she tells her old sweetheart, and became infected.

"Give me a kiss, my love," she asks.

He pecks at her forehead. She tells him in triumph, "I slept with as many of them as I could."

He recoils.

"Why are you so, my love? I have given my life for my country. *I* should have the Military Cross. I killed more of them than you did."

He runs from the hospital. The next day, she dies.

Maupassant lives on. He is solitary but promiscuous. He is a literary success. He likes nothing more than to row on the Seine. Flaubert tells him, fewer whores, less rowing . . . write more stories. Flaubert need not have worried—Maupassant wrote three hundred stories, six novels, three plays, travel books, and poetry.

By 1876, he began to feel "the snake gnawing at his heart," quoting the German poet Heine, who also died from syphilis. Maupassant lost vision in one eye, an event that allowed him to see the "lamentable end."

He is starting to talk wildly, espousing strange thoughts. He writes "Le Horla," the story of a man imperceptibly overtaken by delusions and irrational behavior. At the end of "Le Horla," the man says, "I suppose I must commit suicide." Maupassant complains of worsening migraines that make it difficult for him to write. His memory deteriorates.

"I have without ceasing the horrible sensation of some danger threatening me."

He stops writing.

Maupassant's last sane year is 1891. He travels restlessly and suffers horrendous headaches. He identifies with howling dogs: "Their howling is a lamentable complaint addressed to nobody going nowhere, telling you nothing." He announces that he has been made a count and insists on being recognized as such. In Cannes on New Year's Day, 1892, he tries to kill himself by cutting his throat. He fails. He tries to shoot himself. He fails. The spirochetes multiply in his brain. He becomes delusional and demented.

Guy de Maupassant is taken to the asylum of Dr. Esprit Blanche in a straitjacket. "Monsieur Maupassant is reverting to an animal," says a hospital spokesman to a journalist. He dies on July 6, 1893. His epitaph: "I have coveted everything and taken pleasure in nothing."

On the day of Guy de Maupassant's death, had you walked from Dr. Blanche's sanatorium across the Seine by the Pont de Passy and turned right when you reached the Rue de Vaugirard, a walk of a kilometer, you might have seen, in a lighted room at the corner of the institute bearing his name, Louis Pasteur working in his lab.

THE CAUSATIVE AGENT

Fritz Schaudinn, a lecturer at the University of Berlin, first saw the spirochete through a microscope on March 3, 1905. His friend and colleague Erich Hoffman scraped tissue from a papule on the vulva of a woman with secondary syphilis. Schaudinn saw a spiral-shaped rod, pale and barely visible. He called it *pallidum, Treponema pallidum.*

His finding was rejected at first. Such is the history of science. It is not so surprising when you learn that 125 causes for syphilis had been postulated in the previous twenty years. Schaudinn presented his data to the Berlin Medical Society on May 7, and his evidence could not be resisted. In less than a month, investigators found the treponeme in the liver and spleen of a child who had died of congenital syphilis.

Schaudinn died at age thirty-five the following year from a burst amebic abscess in his abdomen. He had been drinking amebae, experimenting on himself.

The treatment for syphilis in 1905 was the same as it had been in 1606: hot baths, mercury salts, and the holy wood. In 1913, Noguchi Hideyo, the Japanese scientist who was to die fifteen years later in Nigeria of yellow fever he was researching, showed the presence of *Treponema pallidum* in the brain of people who had died of neurosyphilis.

SYPHILIS TODAY

In 2014, an eighteen-year-old man came to see me for medical advice. He had fever, felt ill, noticed swelling of his lymph nodes and a rash over his shoulders. He was well dressed, had just graduated high school, and was waiting to go to college. He was pleasant and cooperative, had not used drugs, had been previously healthy, and was in good general health.

On examination, he had a temperature of 101 degrees Fahrenheit and a pulse rate of 96 per minute. He had a red throat with mild tonsillar swelling and striking enlargement of the lymph nodes of his neck. He was mildly tender over the liver, but the spleen could not be felt. He had a moderate patchy rash, faint and red over his chest and back but not affecting the palms or soles. He told me he had a girlfriend, but they had not been intimate.

"I think I know what this is," I told him. "You have mono."

"That's a relief," he said.

I ordered tests. As a matter of routine, I also ordered an HIV test and then I thought I would throw in an RPR test for syphilis.

In 1942, Howard Florey and Ernst Chain showed that penicillin, discovered in 1928 by Alexander Fleming, was an effective treatment for a number of bacterial infections. In 1944, Dr. John Mahoney, of the Staten Island Marine Hospital Venereal Disease Research Laboratory, decided to give penicillin to four patients with syphilis. In a crowded room, he presented the results, showing rapid recovery in each case. Everyone strained to hear what was being said. One commentator got up to say, "This is probably the most significant paper ever presented in the medical field."

Mahoney was modest. He stated that, "The evaluation of any therapy will require a prolonged trial." But this did not prevent the US Army from quickly introducing penicillin as routine treatment for syphilis. At last, the global scourge was curable. A full human lifetime has elapsed since Mahoney's discovery and no resistant strains of syphilis to penicillin have yet been found.

Two days after seeing the young man described above, I got a call from the New York State lab.

"Hi, Doc. Phew, what a blowout. It's a record."

"What?"

"Mr X. The RPR."

"What about it?"

"Record high. I'll fax you the result."

It was positive 1: 2048.

His mono tests were negative, as was the HIV test. Other sexually transmitted diseases were excluded. There was no doubt—he had secondary syphilis. The lab said they hadn't seen a positive result outside of the city for two years. Our patient hadn't been in the city. There was another contradiction in his story.

Contact tracing is the law of the state in every case of syphilis. My patient's lover was easily found—he was in jail. The details of this liaison were not pursued. Not by me, at any rate. All I cared about was that they were treated. They were given penicillin and cured.

There had been an outbreak of syphilis in New York City in 1988 in tandem with the AIDS epidemic. It occurred at the same time as the street drug of choice changed from heroin to crack cocaine. Heroin is a drug of introspection, opium dens, and nodding; cocaine leads to high frisky, risky behavior. This is yet another example of how epidemics are culturally formed by social attitudes and human behavior.

The incidence of primary, secondary, and congenital syphilis is rising in every state of the United States and all around the world. There were thirteen million new global cases of syphilis in 2019 according to WHO statistics. More than a million sexually transmitted diseases are acquired every day worldwide. Both genital herpes and syphilis increase the risk of contracting HIV infection.

It is seventy-five years since penicillin became the cure for syphilis. The infinite malady has not gone from the world.

CHAPTER 8

FEVER ALL THROUGH
THE NIGHT: MALARIA

B uilt in 1482 by Portuguese adventurer/mariners on the Gold Coast of Africa, Elmina Fort, in Ghana, also known as Elmina Castle, remains, in 2020, the oldest European building south of the Sahara Desert. The Portuguese came for gold (which they found), but they also found the slave trade (which was more profitable).

They were also infected with malaria for the first time.

From the 15th to the 19th centuries, eleven million African slaves were shuttled through waiting stations for transportation across the Atlantic, the Middle Passage, to the Americas and slavery, and 1.8 million passed through the waiting station of Elmina.

Columbus sailed west ten years after Elmina Fort was built. He took infectious diseases with him, to which the indigenous population of Hispaniola and beyond had no resistance—they were a virgin population and were devastated by European diseases.

On the Gold Coast, it was the other way round: indigenous people had the advantage. The Portuguese died from malaria, yellow fever, dysentery, and other infections. They were immunological virgins and were worse off than newborn African babies, who at least had maternal antibodies (and high levels of Hemoglobin F, a type of hemoglobin that protects against malaria) to protect them during their first year of life. Adult Africans were also relatively immune to these infections. If you survived your first one, you then had antibodies—which prevented a further infection or made subsequent illness milder.

MALARIA, COLONIALISTS, AND MISSIONARIES

Malaria is not caused by a bacteria or a virus. It is caused by a protozoan called *Plasmodium* that is injected into the human bloodstream by female *Anopheles* mosquitos. *Plasmodia* feed on blood, and the human body reacts to this invasion with an abrupt onset of high fever with shaking chills. Sometimes the fever comes and goes; sometimes it persists. Nausea, abdominal pain, and diarrhea are frequent symptoms. Low glucose in the blood may occur, particularly in children, which is a danger to the brain. Children are especially vulnerable to malaria infection. In most cases, the spleen enlarges and stays that way so that, in later life, moderate or minor trauma may rupture it.

While the majority recover from malaria, some, especially those with imperfect immunity, suffer lethal complications such as kidney failure, blackwater fever caused by breakage of the red blood cells, brain damage, and secondary bacterial infection. Pregnant women are at least ten times more vulnerable to malaria than non-pregnant women and suffer spontaneous abortion and stillbirth as well as increased mortality of the mother. Immunity comes with survival.

In Elmina, after the Portuguese came the Dutch, and then the British, who, in 1860, hoisted the Union flag over the fort, twenty-seven years after they had abolished slavery. Still, over the next thirty years, as many as two million Africans were rounded up and sent to Cuba and Brazil in spite of a fruitless British blockade. By 1890, these two countries also outlawed slavery, bringing an end to the West African slave trade. The Union flag was taken down on March 6, 1957, and the independent country of Ghana was born.

In these four hundred years of stuttering colonialism, West Africa became known as the White Man's Grave. Because of malaria, the land could not be "settled" as it was in South Africa or in the American colonies, but that didn't stop anyone from trying. In April 1792, 269 British set sail to build a colony on Bolama Island off Guinea Bissau. By November 1793, all but nine had died. Three governors of Sierra Leone died between 1826 and 1828.

In 1832, MacGregor Laird went on a voyage of exploration up the Benue River in what is now Nigeria. Forty of forty-nine Europeans in the expedition died, mostly of fever. The aim had been to convince local tribes to stop slaving as well as to convert them to Christianity. This enterprise was considered so important that a second expedition followed two years later. Fifty of 150 crew, scientists, and physicians perished. The practice of bloodletting as treatment for fever made mortality much worse.

Missionaries were drawn to West Africa by a culture-bound dream in which *the valleys of the continent were to be dotted with British colonies, trading settlements and mission stations, the natives transformed into intelligent, industrious laborers, the valleys blossoming as the rose.* (W. Garden Blakie, *Central Africa Since the Death of Livingstone*, 1897.)

They paid a terrible price for their ill-conceived dream. Whole families—Christian missionary, wife, and children—would make the long sea journey from England to Lagos and die from fever within a week of their arrival. In the three Asante wars of the 19th century, 70 percent of British soldiers fell sick from fever, about a third of whom died. Deaths in combat were 1 percent. As the Asante said, "The white man brings his cannon to the bush, but the bush is stronger than his cannon."

Medical missionary and explorer David Livingstone died from dysentery and malaria in 1873 on the shores of Lake Bangweulu in what is now Zambia. Unfortunately, he did not have access to quinine.

When the medication quinine was introduced in 1850, survival from malaria improved. Missionaries gained greater confidence, and at Westminster there was more talk of colonization. One single medicine may have done more to authorize the "Scramble for Africa" at the turn of the century than any other political or religious force.

THE CAUSE OF MALARIA

Protozoa, now named protists, means "first animal." They dominated life on Earth 1.5 billion years ago and lived primarily by eating bacteria. As more sophisticated creatures evolved, many *Plasmodia* developed a parasitic lifestyle in the animals' intestines. With the advent of insects 150 to 200 million years ago, *Plasmodium* evolved to exist in two hosts, a mosquito and a vertebrate.

Plasmodium mutates through seven different phases in its cycle. It becomes, in effect, seven different protists: sporozoite, merozoite, male gametocyte, female gametocyte, exflagellated microgametocyte, ookinete, and oocyst back to sporozoite. It is complex and beautiful, or we might think it so if it were not eating our blood.

Plasmodia are still doing it. There are hundreds of species, but only six are known, so far, to cause forms of malaria.

Plasmodium falciparum
Plasmodium vivax
Plasmodium ovale Curtis
Plasmodium ovale Walker
Plasmodium malariae
Plasmodium knowlesi

Each has its own characteristics, but we shall only consider the first two. *Plasmodium falciparum* accounts for 99.7 percent of malaria in Africa, 70 percent in Southeast Asia, the Eastern Mediterranean, and the Americas. *Plasmodium vivax*, which barely exists in Africa, accounts for nearly all the rest. Of these six *Plasmodia* of death, *P falciparum* is the most virulent. It was also the last to evolve. This is another example of a general law of plagues, that virulence and recent origin go together. (Just like COVID-19, which will be discussed later.)

Plasmodia only exist as parasites in vertebrates and insects. Their ancestors were algae, a surprising fact, which accounts for the presence of a chloroplast in its cytoplasm, something that is usually only found in plants. Chloroplasts and mitochondria are enslaved bacteria. *Plasmodia* has both. In algae and other green plant cells, the chloroplast is where photosynthesis takes place. There is no photosynthesis in *falciparum*, but the chloroplast persists as it has a specific ability to make isoprene, without which the parasite could not live in the red cells of its hosts.

Plasmodium falciparum jumped into humans from gorillas in Central and West Africa at the beginning of an era called the Holocene, ten thousand years ago, when the Sahara was green. Then it spilled over from us into the bonobo.

Agricultural ideas traveled down into Africa from the Fertile Crescent as the last glacial period came to an end. Hunter-gatherers could see the benefits of communal living along with sowing and reaping. The farmers and the hunters became friends. Humans began living in groups in one place, generating ponds and pools in which the *anopheles* mosquitos could breed. It is estimated that a population of ten thousand people is required for *Plasmodia* to flourish, but other environmental factors such as temperature and the presence of standing water may lower this number.

Arising from still water or marsh, the female of the *anopheles* species injects the protist by feeding in the evening and through the night only. *Aedes aegypti* mosquitos feed twenty-four hours a day. This tiny animal has been killing humans for the last seven thousand years. The greatest mortality is in sub-Saharan Africa, but malaria is also found around the world in a tropical belt from the Indian subcontinent and Southeast Asia to Papua New Guinea, as well as Meso and South America.

Malaria and smallpox are in close competition for being the deadliest diseases in human history. Malaria is certainly our longest-running plague. Between two and three hundred million people lost their lives to malaria in the 20th century alone, accounting for 5 percent of all deaths. In 2019, there were 228 million infections worldwide and 405,000 deaths. Most of these were in sub-Saharan Africa, and 60 percent were children under the age of five.

Falciparum and the slave trade were closely intertwined. After capture inland by Africans in contract with the Europeans, many of the slaves-to-be died on the slow journey to the coast. The cause was rarely malaria. Exhaustion, starvation, and dysentery were more likely. When not walking, they were shackled in crowded, unsanitary *baracoons* or sheds.

The Nigerian American author Adaobi Nwaubani has written about her great-grandfather Nwaubani Ogogo, who was a slave trader. There had been slavery on the African continent for as long as anyone could remember, but the Europeans increased demand. Ogogo would kidnap people from distant villages or sell off prisoners. He sold them, legally, to be transported to Cuba and Brazil. He was a man of some importance and had many wives. When he died, a leopard was killed and six slaves were buried alive with him. He had spiritual powers through the god Njoku. Nwaubani outlines ways in which her generation seeks to atone for the evil of slavery. With the same aim, the Congress of the United States, on June 19, 2019, held a debate on reparations.

Elmina Castle has large dungeons and a door leading to the quay over which was written "A Porta Sem Retorno," the Door of No Return. In these dark and stinking conditions, the enslaved awaited embarkment. Circumstances on board slave ships were as bad or worse as for those held in Elmina. Malnutrition contributed to disease. Yet, from the 18th to the 19th century, mortality among slave traders was higher than that of slaves. Boarding and transporting slaves led to the deaths of one in four slavers, mostly from fever. Eighty per thousand slave deaths was average. They died mostly from flux, aka dysentery. Some jumped overboard. They also suffered from elephantiasis, dropsy, undiagnosed fevers, yaws, and brokenheartedness.

Upon arrival in the United States, there were further health risks, including more travel in chains, dangerous and debilitating work, violent punishment, environmental exposure to European infections, sexual assault and abuse, poor housing, poor sanitation, and inadequate food and clothing. Of the eleven million people transported from Africa, it is estimated that 1.5 million died between capture and arrival at plantations.

The South, home of these plantations, was a primary destination for slaves. Farming tobacco, cotton, and sugarcane were the industries where the slaves were most often wanted. The marshes of the US South were rife with mosquitos and—with the arrival of the slaves and traders who brought it with them—the malaria parasite. The mosquitos came from Africa and established themselves. The protozoa were brought by humans, traders, and slaves until they became endemic.

The traders, the same ones who realized that swollen lymph nodes in the neck was a sign of sleeping sickness, knew that the African slaves' relative immunity to malaria and yellow fever increased their value. They knew that slaves from the Gold Coast, for example, resisted malaria better than those from the Bight of Biafra, so they sold for more.

How did malaria become endemic in the United States? The same way it did in the West Indies and in Brazil and other South American countries. Through the slave trade. The mosquitos brought to the Americas by the slave trade were *anopheles*, *Aedes aegypti*, and *Aedes albopictus*.

Infections Carried to the Americas by the Slave Trade

Malaria isn't the only disease that made the Middle Passage from Africa to the Americas. Others include:

Yellow Fever
Hepatitis B
Hepatitis C
Leprosy
Yaws
Smallpox
HTLV1 Tropical Spastic Paraparesis
Dengue
Chikungunya

The form of malaria called *Plasmodium vivax* is milder than the other common form, *falciparum*, but it is not a mild disease. Unlike *falciparum*, it leaves hypnozoites in the liver. If not properly treated, these sleeping remnants can reactivate months or years after the original infection, causing recurrent bouts of malaria.

Plasmodium vivax also originated in Africa, in chimpanzees and gorillas. It jumped into man and then spread around the world. It has been in existence much longer than *falciparum*. It was infecting *Homo erectus* before *sapiens* appeared. Our ancestors took this heirloom down the Nile and across the Sahara to the Mediterranean. It spread as far north as what is now Denmark. It spread eastward to India and around the world in epidemics that became endemic. Its presence in the Americas before the arrival of Columbus raises the possibility that it was carried over the Bering

Land Bridge. Some have controversially suggested that it was taken there by *Homo erectus* before *sapiens* reached the continent.

When the colonizers arrived, they repeatedly brought fresh cargoes of *Plasmodium*, DNA analysis of which shows that both *falciparum* and *vivax* were brought to South America on slave ships. In South America, 2.7 million people are infected per year, half of those in Brazil.

Bad air circulating from the Pontine Marshes in Italy gave the disease its name, *mal'aria*—bad air. Tooth pulp DNA studies on skeletal remains show that both *falciparum* and *vivax* were prominent two thousand years ago in Italy, and they played their part in the downfall of the Roman Empire. The Emperor Vespasian died of the disease. Malaria was prevalent throughout Europe until fairly recent times. The last Italian *authoctonous* case was in 1962. It may be worth pointing out that the Fontana di Trevi is an excellent breeding ground for mosquitos.

TALES FROM THE SWAMP, PART 1

I was told the new patient in the Emergency Room was forty-eight years old. He spoke Portuguese and one of his female companions interpreted.

"He is herb doctor."

"When did he get here?"

"He left Brazil two days ago and got fever on the plane. And he was shaking like this." She demonstrated.

He looked sick, sure enough. He was ashen, sweating, and perhaps a little breathless. His temperature was 103 degrees Fahrenheit and his pulse was 105 per minute. There was tenderness over the liver and the tip of his spleen could be felt.

"He is herb doctor," she said again. "He is the number one guest speaker at our conference in Woodstock."

"Tell him he has malaria."

He recognized the word and threw up his arms in the air in exasperation.

"He knows. He told us he has malaria. It is common where he comes from. He says he doesn't want American medicines."

"Where does he come from?"

"He is from the Kaxinawa tribe. He comes to Manaus and São Paulo, but he lives with his people. He is pajé, a witch doctor!"

"His name is Bernardo, right?"

"You can call him Bernardo. He says it is his slave name. His real name, he says, is . . . I can't pronounce it."

"Okay, please tell him the blood slide shows *Plasmodium falciparum* malaria—the dangerous kind. We agree with him that he needs herbal treatment. We would like to give him Qinghaso made from the sweet wormwood plant that grows in China."

She starts talking to "Bernardo" in Portuguese. His hair is braided. He has symmetrical abstract tattoos on his arms and torso.

"Doctor, he says he knows Qinghaso, but he prefers tree hide."

"Oh, okay. We will give him tree hide."

"You have it?"

"Yes."

"Bernardo says, how do you prepare the tree hide?"

"Okay, tell him we take a piece of Peruvian bark, also called fever bark or Jesuit bark, about so big and then we boil it in 300 ccs of tap water in a saucepan with juice from half a lemon, a tablespoon of sugar, and I like to throw in some cilantro. After fifteen minutes, I leave it to simmer for an hour, hour and a half, and then I decant the supernatant fluid and voilà, I have the six doses I need to cure him."

As this is being relayed, Bernardo lies back on the gurney in a posture of exhaustion. In spite of which, he begins to laugh softly, which makes him cough. He reaches out his hands, takes one of mine, and squeezes it laughing and coughing.

"He says he like you. He says he knows you are, excuse me, Doctor, saying bullshit? But he will take your tree hide."

And so, I gave him quinine, 600 mgs, infused over four hours, every eight hours. Slightly less than twenty-four hours later, the patient is much better. He is switched to oral quinine and doxycycline. The physician keeps quiet about the origin of the doxy.

Even "Bernardo" is happy.

I advise him, via interpreter, "Don't take any American medicines with the ones I gave you and don't take any herbs until you are better."

We both smile at the irony.

The bark of the cinchona tree, or Peruvian bark, was discovered to be preventative and curative of malaria. It was the first medicine with this sort of power in use, three hundred years before antibiotics.

"More precious than silver or gold," said Dr. Sebastian Bado in 1650.

"It has the same significance to medicine as gunpowder did to the art of war," opined Professor Bernardino Ramazzini in 1660. "The greatest gift of the new world to the old."

The first to be aware of its powers would have been the indigenous peoples of the Amazon rain forest. In 1620, an indigenous person treated a Jesuit missionary in what is now Loxa, Ecuador, who recovered from his fever. The tree from which the bark comes was named after the Countess of Chinchon, wife to the Viceroy of Peru. She was cured of fever according to legend, and the tree was named after her, although the first "H" was dropped. In the local language it was called the Quina Quina tree. Because it was "discovered" by the Jesuits, it was also known as Jesuit's bark or Jesuit's powder and was therefore very unpopular with Protestants. By 1658, the Jesuit powder had reached China. It became much prized in Europe, and punishment by death was invoked in Peru for anyone trying to steal the seeds of the tree and breaking their monopoly. Nevertheless, botanists stole seeds.

Charles Ledger, in 1856, stole some with high concentration of quinine and sold them to the king of Holland. *Cinchona ledgeriana* trees blossomed with quinine content and so did trade. Trade was sweet; the medicine was bitter. Many believe that a medicine is no good unless it is bitter.

Quinine found another niche in soft drinks—tonic water. Gins and tonics were supposed to ward off malaria and protect colonialists in pith helmets and back pads, just as they wore jackboots to protect themselves from snakes. Each bottle of Indian Tonic Water contains 68 milligrams of quinine. It gives a delicious bitterness also found in the aperitifs Dubonnet and Lillet. However, you'd have to consume five liters daily of any of these to get protection from malaria.

Quinine has been isolated from the bark. It has also been synthesized, yet industrial-scale production does not exist. Quinine is still made by extracting it from the bark of trees that are primarily grown on plantations in the troubled Kivu province of the Democratic Republic of Congo.

When *Plasmodia* get inside the red blood cell, they break down hemoglobin. The globin part of the molecule is full of amino acids, which are nutritious, but the heme is potentially toxic to the parasite so they crystallize the heme, rendering it harmless. Quinine stops this crystallization, sounding the protozoan's death knell.

TALES FROM THE SWAMP, PART 2

Ethiopian Airlines Flight 900 took off from Murtala Muhammed Airport in Lagos bound for Stockholm, Sweden, via Addis Ababa. It is August 2005. There is at least one mosquito aboard. She probably ate on the plane. Sixteen hours later, at six in the morning, as soon as the hatch opened at Arlanda Airport in Sweden, she flew away into the cold summer air of the north.

She managed to fly in through a small opening of the driver's-side window of the Volvo Johan Johannsen was driving near the airport. She sat on his neck and extended her proboscis to pierce his skin. The proboscis is made of two parallel tubes. It sends saliva down the outer tube, which helps pump blood up the inner tube. The saliva contains a blood thinner and, of course, malarial sporozoites waiting in her salivary glands. She squirted and drank for about three minutes. She drank about a milliliter of blood and injected seventy-five sporozoites into his bloodstream.

Shortly afterwards, she perished in the northern air.

Johan is driving to Jokkmokk in Swedish Lapland, which is 635 miles away and north of the Arctic Circle. He expects the trip to take at least twelve hours. He is going to meet his girlfriend, Maja, there, who is working at the summer market. He feels fine, yet the sporozoites have already made their way into his liver cells. They start to multiply. They will multiply up to thirty thousand times before the onset of symptoms—four to seven days after the bite. After about half an hour, he feels an itchy spot on his neck and scratches it absentmindedly. He is blissfully unaware that exoerythrocytic schizogony is underway in his liver.

About a week later, he feels tired. Because it is summer, it is light pretty much all the time, but at 7:30 PM he tells Maja that he is going to bed early, takes aspirin, and sleeps. At 1:00 AM, he wakes up and vomits once.

At three o'clock, he wakes again because he is shaking. The bed is jiggling so much with his shaking chills that Maja also wakes up. She takes Johan's temperature and it is 41 degrees Centigrade, which is nearly 106 Fahrenheit. She gives him more aspirin. "I must have the flu," he says. In reality, the merozoites that have colonized and multiplied in his red blood cells are rupturing them. This is the asexual erythrocytic phase. He shakes for a full forty-five minutes. He feels very unwell and starts to sweat profusely. A few hours later, he suffers another episode of shaking chills and has a bout of diarrhea. *I must have gastroenteritis*, he thinks. And here we come to a critical question. Which doctor in Jokkmokk, north of the Arctic Circle, is going to diagnose malaria in a man from Stockholm who has never left the country?

Airport malaria, also known as suitcase malaria, is rare but increasing in incidence. About one hundred patients have been reported, but there is always underreporting. With air travel, imported malaria is more frequent due to the patient traveling from a malaria-endemic country during the incubation period. There are ninety-one countries endemic for malaria, and each year there are about two thousand cases reported in the US, at least one in every state. Twice as many were reported in both France and the UK. Nigeria and other West African countries are the origin in a third of cases but they may come from any country where the disease is endemic.

An important group to recognize and educate before they travel are those raised in a malaria endemic zone, for example those born in Ghana who have been at school or employed for a year or two in the UK or the US. Over the course of about two years, they will lose their partial, but significant, immunity. When they travel back home, they are like one-year-old infants again, as far as their immunity to malaria is concerned. They don't take preventative antimalarials. They never did growing up—why should they start now? Such people are at high risk.

Caught up in these statistics are cryptic cases that are attributable neither to mosquitos flying in on a plane nor to humans importing the disease. Most of these are probably airport malaria. How else could a Swede suddenly develop malaria north of the Arctic Circle?

So, what happened to Johan Johannsen? Maja insisted he go to the hospital, which is always a good first step. The doctors were predictably mystified. A number of curious and rare diseases were proposed as the cause of his illness. Yet there was good fortune in the eagle eye of the lab technologist looking at Johan's blood film. He drew the doctors' attention to the strange little spots inside the patient's red blood cells.

Johannsen is ultimately treated with quinine. Treat first, ask questions later. He recovers.

A child dies of malaria every thirty seconds in the world. Why is this disease still with us? The life cycle is understood, we know how to prevent it, and although some strains have developed resistance to some antimalarials, we have effective treatment. This preventable, treatable disease infected 228 million people worldwide in 2019 and led to the deaths of 405,000, with *Plasmodium falciparum* responsible for most.

It is true that over the last decade there has been an improvement in these statistics, but with the advent of resistant strains, population explosion, the growth of megalopolises such as Kinshasa and Mumbai, together with poverty and poor control measures due to bad government, this improvement is stalling. The consequences are not merely the death of children. Infection with malaria weakens resistance to other infections such as measles. It entrenches and worsens poverty. It degrades infrastructure and increases costs.

In her book *The Fever*, the journalist Sonia Shah points out not only the challenge of poverty but also of cultural blockades. The paradox is that those who live in malaria zones are the ones who care least about it. For them, it's a normal problem of life. Wole Soyinka, the Nobel laureate in literature, flew to a meeting in Switzerland, bringing fever with him. When he was told he had malaria, he discharged himself from the hospital saying,

> When people back home hear that Wole Soyinka was kept in hospital because of . . . MALARIA! I will be stripped of my nationality, my passport will be taken away and people will drive around my house with empty tin cans strung to the backs of their cars. I will be the laughingstock of the nation. And you know why? Because we in Nigeria have malaria for breakfast lunch and dinner.

So, how do you get anyone to do something about malaria when the people don't seem to mind? At the same time, outsiders recommending mosquito nets and insecticides have also failed. The desire to eradicate must come from within.

There is some (fairly) good news. There is a vaccine being studied by the WHO in a pilot program in Malawi, Kenya, and Ghana. It will continue through 2023.

Man's ingenuity will be strained to the utmost to find a vaccine for a protozoa that metamorphoses and survives seven times in a cold-blooded insect and a warm-blooded vertebrate, both of which are trying to suppress it. We await the results expectantly.

Also holding promise is the introduction into the world of genetically modified mosquitos that cannot be infected. There goes Man interfering with Nature again.

CHAPTER 9

INVISIBLE KILLERS:
VIRUSES

Viruses are the leading killers of humans—more than war, famine, and bacterial pestilence put together. The death count is in the high hundreds of millions. The word comes from the Latin, meaning *slimy poison*, and had been in use a long time before it acquired its modern sense in the late 19th century.

Most viruses are one hundred thousandth the width of a human hair. Yet, if all the viruses in the world were placed one on top of one another, they would reach 200 million light-years into space. As astonishing as this sounds, it may be an understatement. We live and flourish in clouds of viruses. We breath them in on a daily basis. We eat 10^9 viruses per gram of salad. Fortunately, plant viruses do not cause infection in humans and we excrete the same number that we eat.

Wherever you have life, you have viruses, as they are the most abundant biological entity on the planet. If you go into the rain forest, which teems with life, there are more viruses than anywhere else except the ocean. There are currently 8.7 million species of plants and animals that have been identified. If we estimate there are ten viruses per species, that comes to eighty-seven million species of virus. To date, we have documented the existence of 4,404, although the number has certainly gone up since this sentence was written. This means that 99.994 percent of virus species are currently unidentified. Of those that have been documented in humans and are capable of causing disease, there are 219 viruses and counting.

A virus is an infective agent that consists of either a DNA or an RNA core surrounded by a protein coat. There is more DNA, that is, genetic information, in bacteria than in animals and plants combined. There is more DNA in viruses than animals, plants, *and* bacteria combined. Viruses are metabolically inert and can only replicate in living cells. Sounds problematic for their survival, doesn't it? On the contrary, the number of viruses on Earth is 10^{33}, which is a billion times more than a trillion trillion.

When viruses infect, they enter cells, take over the mechanism of replication, and churn out copies of themselves until the cell bursts. Then they enter new cells to replicate further. Pretty soon you're talking billions of copies.

VIRUSES, DEAD OR ALIVE?

Viruses are a conundrum. They are not alive. They can only replicate in the cells of other organisms. They can kill an elephant. They have caused the worst pandemics in human history, including smallpox, AIDS, and COVID-19. Yet, they are not dead. They are not inanimate in the sense that a stone is inanimate. Perhaps they are alive when replicating in a cell, and that which we call a virus is an intermediate spore-like entity. Outside the cell they are a chemical, and inside the cell they are biological. They exist on a spectrum between not alive and living. Call them replicators.

They have the same DNA or RNA that all living things have. Feels odd, doesn't it, to know that we share the world with trillions upon trillions of creatures so small most of them can't be seen through a light microscope? And their genes are made of the same DNA as ours.

In the beginning of life on Earth, three and a half billion years ago, ribonucleic acid (RNA) formed in hydrothermal vents deep in the oceans. It was the first biological molecule to store genetic information as well as catalyzing its own replication. This was the RNA world. The simplest infectious form of nucleic acid is RNA found in viroids. Viroids are noncoding RNA and do not have a protein coat (a characteristic of viruses). Nevertheless, they have virus-like properties and in modern times cause substantial disease in plants. There is only one viroid known to cause disease in humans so far: delta virus hepatitis. However, delta virus can only cause infection in a liver cell that is already infected with Hepatitis B Virus. RNA viruses are a step up in complexity from viroids. They have a protein coat and code for specific amino acids, the building blocks of proteins. RNA viruses are some of the most dangerous to *H sapiens*. The Baltimore classification of viruses is a system that groups them according to the type of nucleic acid each species has. There are eight categories, three with RNA alone.

When RNA replicates, it makes many "mistakes," which is another way of saying its structure changes rapidly. Some of these changes are beneficial to its life cycle. In other words, it *evolves* rapidly, sometimes up to a million times faster than the host it is infecting.

It is not in the interest of a pathogen to kill its host. If it does, it kills itself. It can circumvent this fate by being transmitted to another individual, either of the same species or another. The evolution of these viruses allows rapid adaptation to a new host.

Other viruses become less lethal to survive. RNA viruses are so good at adapting to the new host that there is less need to blunt their virulence. This explains why RNA viruses are some of the most lethal known to man. Ebola. Rabies. HIV and, yes, SARS-CoV-2. They are all relics of the primordial RNA world.

Of all protein-synthesizing replicating entities, that is, *life*, on Earth, only these three classes of viruses use RNA to code their protein information. Every other life form uses DNA. DNA is more stable, allowing for much larger genomes than RNA viruses. In the DNA world, protein enzymes perform the necessary catalytic tasks with far greater efficiency than RNA catalyzes itself. RNA still produces fundamental reactions in modern-day cells. If DNA is the library book, RNA is the piece of paper on which the message is scribbled.

VIROLOGY

In 1892, Dmitri Ivanovsky showed that *tobacco mosaic blight* could be transferred to healthy plants by mashing up unhealthy plants and passing them through a porcelain filter whose pores were too small to allow bacteria to pass. Martinus Beijerinck, a contemporary Dutch plant microbiologist, confirmed this work and called the transmitting factor a virus. Although their work appeared to be only of interest to botanists, these humble plant experiments were the beginning of the science of virology, with vast implications for the past and particularly the future of the human race.

The first human disease conclusively shown to be caused by a virus was yellow fever in 1927, followed by influenza in 1931. It is remarkable that we knew anything at all about viruses (not to mention their link to disease) before the first electron microscope was developed in 1932. Knowledge of viral structure followed the elucidation of the structure of the DNA molecule in 1953. The arrival of the computer allowed large amounts of data about viruses to be more easily interrogated. This way we have learned more about viruses in the last ten years than in all human history. We are living in the Golden Age of Virology.

THE HUMAN GENOME PROJECT

By 2003, the Human Genome Project completed the sequence of a human genome over eight years at the cost of $2.7 billion. It was three billion base pairs long and it is one of the most fruitful scientific achievements ever undertaken.

The first draft was published in *Nature* in February 2001, and it immediately presented two surprising truths. The first was that only 1.5 percent of the genes sequenced were responsible for the 21,000 body proteins that make up our structure and metabolism. The second was that we are made up of genes from many different sources. There is 5 percent from fungi, 20 to 30 percent from bacteria, and nearly 50 percent from *viruses*. Yes, you are half virus. These are *endogenous* viruses of a select group known as retroviruses.

RETROVIRUSES AND ENDOGENOUS RETROVIRUSES

In 1982, Anthony Gallo of the National Cancer Institute in Washington, DC, described the first retrovirus to cause disease in humans, the *human*

T cell lymphotropic virus (HTLV 1). At that time, AIDS was sweeping the world. Its cause, the *human immunodeficiency virus (HIV)*, was discovered by Luc Montagnier and Francoise Barré-Sinoussi in Paris in 1984 and, remarkably, it was also a retrovirus, the second shown to cause human disease.

What is a retrovirus? A retrovirus has the ability to integrate its nucleic acid into the nuclear DNA of the cell it infects. It enters the cell through a receptor on the cell's surface in the usual way. It carries a single strand of RNA that is converted into double-stranded DNA by an enzyme, reverse transcriptase, for which it carries the code. The virus then integrates itself into the cell's nuclear DNA. From there the structure of a new retrovirus is replicated over and over again, the viral parts reassembling in the cytoplasm of the cell to bud out into the bloodstream until it attaches to other cells. The retroviral DNA integrated into the cell's DNA remains there.

If the cell being infected by a retrovirus is an ovum or a sperm, retroviral DNA can be transmitted to the next generation and subsequent generations for as long as the species survives. That is how retroviruses, now called endogenous retroviruses, come to be in your genome. Has this happened often? There are remnants of 98,000 human endogenous retroviruses (HERVs) classified into thirty families making up 8 percent of your genome. They can no longer produce virus particles. They have been accumulating in vertebrates for ten million years and are also referred to as fossil viruses.

The retroviruses in our genome have caused evolutionary change. It is possible that we might have been a very different species without them. For example, the development of the placenta in mammals depends on proteins produced by endogenous retroviruses that entered the mammalian genome twenty-five million years ago. The placenta could not have evolved without a retroviral protein called *syncytin*. Without the placenta, human beings would be laying eggs.

The impact of endogenous retroviral proteins remains underestimated. There is a protein from a retrovirus called ARC that allows RNA in brains to travel from one neuron to the next. This plays a critical role in learning and other cognitive processes. Dysfunction of ARC may lead to Alzheimer's disease, autism, and other disorders of impaired cognition. It is startling to note that brain power, that which we admire most about ourselves, is dependent upon a protein first synthesized in a virus.

Lastly, endogenous retroviruses inhibit entry into the cell of other viruses, conferring a powerful component of immunity. Of the known-to-date retroviruses that cause disease in *Homo sapiens* (HIV1, HIV2, and HTLVI), there is no evidence that they have entered the germ line via sperm or ovum. So far.

MIMIVIRUS

In 1993, in the North of England, researchers discovered a "bacterium" in amebae that didn't follow the rules. Unlike typical bacteria, it couldn't be cultured and it wouldn't stain. It took ten years to realize this was because the organism was a virus, leading to a revision of the definition of a virus. Previously, viruses had been defined as being filter-passing agents that could not be seen under the light microscope. These entities were filtered and *could* be seen under a light microscope. So, they were named microbe mimicking virus, or *mimivirus*. No longer regarded with incredulity, there are one hundred species and counting of mimiviruses that have been detected all over the world, from Australia to the Amazon. Many infect amebae, which are found in cooling towers, air conditioners, ponds, and puddles. Other mimiviruses infect plankton in the ocean. They have been around for 2.7 billion years. The genome of mimiviruses is always made of double-stranded DNA, and a typical organism will have 500,000 base pairs. For comparison, influenza virus has 13,588 base pairs in its genome.

OCEANS, VIRUSES, AND LIFE ITSELF

One aspect of viruses is straightforward. They cause about 200 diseases. These little demons from hell get inside us, cause infections that make us sick, kill us directly, or cause cancer (Hepatitis B, HIV, Epstein-Barr). Me, you, our families, our children, our friends . . . we are all susceptible.

Wait a minute, says Karin Moelling, eminent virologist and author of *Viruses: More Friends Than Foes*. This definition is medically biased. There are 10^{33} viruses on the planet and only 10^9 humans. *We are invaders in their world*, she writes. *They only cause disease when an equilibrium gets out of balance.*

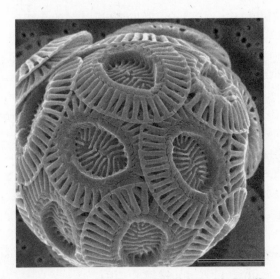

Emiliana huxleyi, *plankton alga covered with coccoliths. Alison R. Taylor (University of North Carolina Wilmington Microscopy Facility), CC BY 2.5.*

Every quart of seawater contains up to one hundred billion viruses. An accidental sip while swimming at Coney Island or Virginia Beach contains a hundred million to a billion viruses, primarily those that infect bacteria, known as bacteriophage or phage. They rarely do humans any harm. In the sea, 98 percent by weight of all living matter is viral, mostly phage. Fully 80 percent are novel organisms, unknown to science, representing an enormous biological diversity. If you put all the viruses of the oceans on a scale, they would weigh the equivalent of seventy-five million blue whales. Every day, viruses kill about half of all bacteria in the world's oceans. Every second, ten trillion bacteria are infected. The latest evidence suggests there are two hundred thousand species of virus in the ocean, from the surface down to four thousand meters and from the North to the South Pole.

Viruses transfer a trillion, trillion genes between host genomes in the ocean every year. This shuttling of genes has had a huge impact on the history of life on Earth. It was in the oceans that life got its start, after all.

We are dependent on bacteria for oxygen. Half of the world's oxygen is produced by plants as a by-product of photosynthesis. The other half comes from cyanobacteria and blue-green algae in the oceans. In many cases, cyanobacteria acquired the genes for photosynthesis from viral infections, and in some cases the viruses augment the production of oxygen. One estimate says that 10 percent of the world's oxygen comes from viral genes. One in every ten breaths is thanks to viruses.

Viruses also clean up the ocean. They disperse algal blooms, also known as red and green tides. *Emiliana huxleyi* (Ehux) is one of the most abundant planktons in the ocean. Found everywhere except in the polar seas, it belongs to the family Coccolithophores, organisms surrounded by little plates of calcium carbonate. In favorable conditions, Ehux aggregates into massive blooms as large as England and visible to space satellites. They may be infected by a number of viruses, particularly the mimivirus coccolithovirus. When Ehux plankton is infected and killed, calcium carbonate falls to the bottom of the sea. Over millions of years and with changes in sea levels, the sediment becomes chalk cliffs.

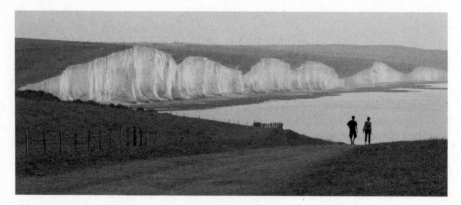

Image credit Edward Dalmulder. Seven Sisters, East Sussex, England.

When you stand on cliffs, you are actually standing on the sediment of countless chalky shells of Ehux killed by giant viruses over the course of millions of years. The smell of the ocean comes from the chemical dimethyl sulfide, released by the lysis (disintegration) of algae by viruses. Lighter parts of the shell, freed after its lysis by viruses, rise in the air as an aerosol, affecting cloud creation, formation, and movement, and ultimately causing downpours.

A couple stands on a chalk cliff gazing out to sea. They smell the sea breeze and look up at the ever-changing clouds. They know nothing of viruses. It begins to rain.

CHAPTER 10

....

THE GODDESS
IN RED: SMALLPOX

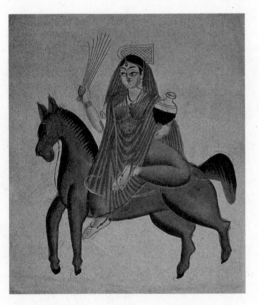

Sitala.

The Hindu goddess Sitala wears a red-colored dress, rides a donkey, and carries the seeds of lentils. She is also the goddess of *masurica*, now called *basanta roga* and known in the English-speaking world as smallpox. She can both cause it and cure it. Sitala was created by Lord Brahma, and he promised that she would be worshipped as a goddess on Earth. Sitala demanded supremacy over all other gods, and when a mortal king refused to worship her, she spread pox on the land by turning lentils, *masurica*, into smallpox. Sitala also means "the cool one," based on her ability to cool high fevers. She is indifferent to caste. Celebrations of the goddess are the only times untouchables, *harijaan*, are allowed into the village temple. Sitala's companion is Djvarasura, whose name means "fever demon." He was created from the sweat on the forehead of the meditating Shiva, and was killed by the god Vishnu, who cut him into three pieces. Djvarasura was revived by Brahma who rejoined the three parts, each of which had grown a head and limbs. Djvarasura moves in every direction at once; what better symbol for a pandemic disease could be found? He became the consort of the smallpox goddess. They travel on the same donkey, with him disguised as a young servant.

That must have been some disguise.

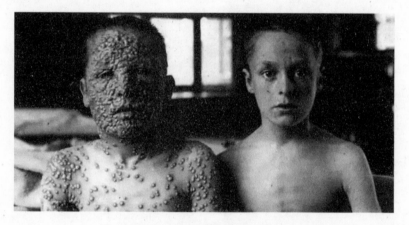

One boy has been vaccinated, one not.
Photograph taken circa 1901 by Dr. Allan Warner.

PANDEMIC

In 1757, at the Battle of Plassey, Robert Clive defeated the twenty-year-old Nawab of Bengal, leading to British domination of the Indian subcontinent for the next two hundred years. After the battle, a string of unimaginable misfortunes followed.

Crops failed, drought followed, and then plagues followed the drought—smallpox, malaria, typhus, typhoid, cholera, influenza, and tuberculosis. An estimated ten million people lost their lives in this catastrophe. All were afflicted equally; status was no protection. The new Nawab of Bengal contracted smallpox two weeks after his coronation and died. His brother was crowned only to die two weeks later from the same disease. The pandemic swept through India. Land that had been cultivated returned to the jungle. Bands of bandits, *Thugee*, roamed the country.

Inoculation, also known as variolation, had been practiced in India for a thousand years. The skin is pricked and then rubbed with a small wad of cotton with matter from smallpox scabs saved from the previous year mixed with a drop or two of Ganges water. Inoculation was known in several cultures as a folk remedy. The trouble was that it wasn't widely practiced. Many Hindus refused to interfere in the domain of Sitala, and Muslims were strongly resistant because there is no mention of inoculation in the Holy Quran.

Hindu priests would advise:

Whoever afflicted by fever should say, 'O Sitala Sitala!' and his dreadful fear of pustules immediately vanishes.
O Sitala, for a man scorched by fever, become foul smelling, and whose vision is destroyed, you they regard as the living medicine.
I bow down to Sitala Devi.

~Hymn to Sitala, 16th century

For two hundred years through the 19th and 20th centuries, the subcontinent and its neighbors, now known as Sri Lanka, Myanmar, Vietnam, Afghanistan, and Iran, were scourged by *masurica* every five to ten years with appalling mortality, human suffering, and sociological consequences.

Variola major, its scientific name, has killed 300 million people in the 20th century alone and 600 million since the first known outbreak. It is first on any list of the microbes that have hurt us. Its history is intimately intertwined with the world's history. It was also the first pandemic disease for which a successful vaccine was manufactured and the first and only plague in humans eradicated from the earth.

The origin of the virus is unclear. It is likely that it jumped from the camel or the *sole-jerbil* to *Homo sapiens* between 16,000 and 68,000 years ago. Viruses from these animals have DNA that is closer to the human variola virus than any other yet discovered, including cowpox. Perhaps the domestication of camels along the northeast coast of Africa was the origin of this particular devastation. The virus reached pandemic levels as towns and cities developed because it requires a minimum population size to continue replicating. Once it has that, it becomes highly contagious, and it spread to every country in the world.

Through close personal contact, the virus is inhaled and, after an incubation period of seven to twenty-two days, a high fever and a diffuse, smooth rash develops. This is the prodrome. Three days later, it is replaced by a rash all over the body with papules filled at first with clear fluid that is replaced with cloudy fluid. They appear on the arms, legs, hands, and feet rather than on the torso. Fresh crops of pustules appear as others fade. As the rash appears, the fever disappears. The sick give off an unpleasant odor. About 30 percent of infected people die—more if their health has been compromised by malnutrition or other disease. Smallpox progresses to shock, bleeding into the skin, clotting of veins, delirium, and death. Survivors are at risk for blindness, scarring of the face and body, baldness, loss of eyebrows, infertility or sterility, and arthritis, not to mention psychiatric issues. Pregnant women have a higher mortality and suffer greatly increased risk of spontaneous abortion and still-birth. Although smallpox originated in other mammals, it has adapted to humans uniquely.

The reward for survival is permanent immunity.

The last two people on Earth to get smallpox, so far, were Janet Parker and her mother. In 1978, Janet was a forty-two-year-old medical photographer at the University of Birmingham, England. Her office was directly above a lab where Professor Henry Bedson was studying the virus. She thought she had a cold and then came the telltale rash. She was quarantined along with her parents. Her mother got a fever; it was smallpox. Then her father suffered an unexpected heart attack and died. Bedson committed suicide—it is thought out of guilt. Janet died on the seventh day of her illness. Her mother recovered.

Although smallpox has been eradicated, Russia, America, and possibly others maintain samples of the virus for potential use as biological weapons.

FIGHTING SMALLPOX

As we saw from the salutary Indian practice mentioned earlier, material from a smallpox pustule rubbed into a small, self-inflicted wound usually leads to a mild disease, giving immunity for life. In China, blowing powdered scab into a nostril has the same effect. Left nostril for boys, right nostril for girls. These approaches worked well, except that 5 percent of people given either method died from smallpox.

RED THERAPY

One of many folk remedies for the disease, the color red as therapy was widely used against smallpox. Sitala wears a red dress. Nyang Nyang, a Chinese goddess, insisted that the first pustules were to be swabbed with red pigment, and patients should wear a red cloth on their head as they appeared before a figure of the goddess. A red gourd would be hung out of the window to treat, warn others, and serve as a receptacle for scabs.

In Japan, clothes, toys, and sweets must be red, and a picture of Tametomo, a famous archer painted in red, was hung in sickrooms to speed recovery. Should the child start to recover, a small piece of red cloth would be put on his or her head. The smallpox devils, *hosogami*, feared the color. This association was not confined to the Far East. The medieval Mediterranean physicians Avicenna and Averroes both recommended red in the form of red clothes and red medicines to treat smallpox.

Gilbert the Englishman in his monumental medical text, the *Compendium Medicinae*, wrote in 1240 that red artifacts were beneficial in treating smallpox. He recounts how country women gave purple or red drinks to those with the spotted disease.

John of Gaddesen, in England a hundred years later, cured King Edward II's son by wrapping him completely in red cloth and making everything around his bed red. Prince John was made to suck a red pomegranate and to gargle mulberry wine.

In 1562, Elizabeth the First, Queen of England, was taken ill with a high fever. She survived smallpox after a worrying course. She was wrapped twice daily in a red body cloth. She lost her eyebrows and her hair. She was not too badly pocked in the face, unlike her friend and nurse, Lady Mary Sidney, who was terribly disfigured. Sidney's husband had left "a full fayre ladye in myne eye at least the fairest. When I returned she was as fowle as the Small Pox could make her. She was like a night raven in the house."

Turks in the 18th century draped red cloth around a patient's bed, and red rags were used to wrap around the arm of the inoculated child.

Sopona, also Babalu Aye, are names for the god of smallpox among the Yoruba of West Africa. He dresses in red, and smallpox is a sign of his divine displeasure. Like Sitala, he brings both disease and its cure. The color is reserved for him and those with the disease.

In the late 19th century, Professor Niels Finsen in Copenhagen treated smallpox with red light. He called it erythrotherapy. He wrote, *The action of light on the course of smallpox is astonishing . . . one of the most striking results known in medicine*. He died in 1904, but his treatment survived him by many years. In 1925, it was still in use in Poland, France, and Rumania.

And then along came science. In 1904, London physicians Ricketts and Byles wrote, *We cannot agree that the red light treatment has any of the merits that have been claimed for it*. In retrospect, the ruddy light was neither more harmful nor more effective than the prevailing treatments of purging and bloodletting.

And still smallpox's scarlet overtone wouldn't fade. I vividly recall during my childhood in the 1950s that English children who had been vaccinated wore a red armband for three days.

SMALLPOX IN BOSTON

Cotton Mather was a Bostonian, the last of the Puritans. In 1721, smallpox struck his city. It wouldn't be the only time. There were sixteen significant epidemics in Boston over the next 180 years, the last being 1901–1903.

This was the first pandemic. A sailor arriving from Barbados had been brought ashore from the HMS *Seahorse* with fever and spots. He was quickly isolated, but several shipmates fell ill and the disease spread swiftly. Men were quarantined in a harbor house with a red flag and a sign that said, "God have Mercy on this House."

Cotton Mather strongly advocated inoculation, sparking a controversy that was so intense someone threw a bomb filled with gunpowder and turpentine through his window with a note: "Cotton Mather you dog, damn you, I'll inoculate you with this." The bomb did not explode.

Mather had learned about inoculation from his slave Onesimus, who was born in Burkina Faso, West Africa, and who had never had smallpox. Mather spoke to other Africans who showed him the inoculation scars on their arms. Mather had also read about the practice in Turkey and he may have heard of Lady Mary Wortley Montagu, wife of the British ambassador to Turkey, who popularized inoculation upon return to England. She had had smallpox and it left her without eyebrows and with a pocked face. In 1718, she successfully inoculated her five-year-old son.

The arguments against Mather were vigorous and varied. Inoculation was against Divine Law by countering God's specific will. It was not mentioned in the Bible. Then there was the risk of inflicting harm on innocent people. The most powerful voice raised against Mather was that of Dr. William Douglas who alone of Boston's physicians actually had a medical degree. Douglas feared unchecked inoculation would worsen the epidemic. He asserted that the treatment was untested and based on folklore. In the midst of this controversy, Mather was threatened with hanging. He wrote in his diary, *I never saw the devil so let loose upon any occasion. A lying spirit was gone forth at such a rate that there was no believing anything one heard . . . But never any patients had so many pustules of the small pox, as there were lies now daily told and spread among our deluded people.*

The young Benjamin Franklin, then in Boston, wrote about inoculation in his newspaper, the *New-England Courant*: *It is against God's providence, Most of the ministers are for it and that induces me to think it is the work of the D . . . l, for he often makes use of good men as instruments to obtrude his Delusions on the World.* Years later in Philadelphia, Franklin's young son Franky died of smallpox in 1731, at the age of five, which grieved him bitterly and caused him to regret his anti-inoculation stance.

Those who opposed inoculation had a point. To inoculate was to give an infection. They were contagious, and a small number died from the practice. This methodology wouldn't pass a Research Review Board today.

Dr. Zabdiel Boylston inoculated 287 people, of whom six—or 2 percent—died. Of the un-inoculated, the mortality was 14.8 percent. When the next epidemic arrived in Boston in 1731, Dr. William Douglas acknowledged and practiced inoculation, and its use spread throughout the colonies. George Washington, who had caught and survived smallpox, insisted that his entire army be inoculated. It proved a wise decision by the future president: The death from smallpox in the ranks fell from 17 percent to 1 percent.

EDWARD JENNER

In England, it had been known for a long time that dairymaids were immune to smallpox. In 1774, a dairy farmer from Devon, England, called Jesty, in the middle of a smallpox epidemic, scratched the arms of his wife and two children and rubbed material from a pock on a cow's udder into the scratch. This was the first example of vaccination. It protected his family. When his action became known, he was hooted at and pelted with stones in the marketplace. He was expected to grow horns.

He insisted he was not the first to use this method. Dr. Fewster in 1765 gave a paper entitled "Cow pox and its ability to prevent Smallpox." Fewster didn't think his observation had any value. After all, he reasoned, we already had variolation.

The first person Edward Jenner treated with cowpox was James Phipps, an eight-year-old boy. The donor was the dairymaid Sarah, and the cow was called Blossom. James felt slightly unwell for a day or two. On the ninth day, he was injected with smallpox pus. He didn't get the disease. Happily, James did well and never acquired smallpox. Unhappily, he died as a young man from tuberculosis.

There was no mortality and only rare illness associated with vaccination. It was the mainstay of the elimination of smallpox, first from

England, then Europe, and by 1976, from the earth. No single man has saved as many lives as Edward Jenner.

ANTI-VACCINATION

Despite the success of vaccines, there has always been an international minority opposition to their use that comes from several quarters.

Religious objection: In addition to Hindus not wanting to antagonize Sitala, and Muslims and Protestant Christians refusing variolation as it is not mentioned in the Holy Quran or the Holy Bible, members of the Church of England's hierarchy objected to vaccination because "Fear of smallpox is a happy restraint upon many people . . . to keep themselves in Temperance and Sobriety."

It is harmful or it doesn't work: "It's introducing a bestial humor into the human frame. Poison is taken from a brute creation, of the origin nature and effects of which they had not the smallest knowledge." Biologist Lord Alfred Russel Wallace, the eminent cofounder of natural selection, had a deep opposition and even wrote a book titled *Vaccination a Delusion: Its Penal Enforcement a Crime.* His main complaint was that "it doesn't work."

As vaccination was more widely used, it attracted opposition across Europe. None of the opposition stopped it from being used to the substantial benefit of mankind.

It infringes on the rights of the individual: In 1870, the government of England prescribed vaccination for all or face fines, confiscation of property, or the workhouse. This led to uproar with public demonstrations in a number of British cities. The *Antivaccinator* was published. In response, the law was modified to allow conscientious objection. America had an even more aggressive reaction to vaccination. James Martin Peebles, American physician and spiritualist, wrote the 1900 book *Vaccination a Curse and a Menace to Personal Liberty.* He described vaccination as "the crowning outrage upon the personal liberty of the American Citizen."

It is part of a plot: In 2003, polio immunization officials in Kano State, Nigeria, were murdered following the teaching of Dr. Datti Ahmed that insisted polio immunization was a Western or American scheme to induce infertility in Muslims. In 2012, Taliban spokesman Ehsanullah Ehsan, speaking in the newspaper *Dawn*, said, "It was a conspiracy of Jews and Christians to make Muslims impotent and to stunt their growth." By 2020, the number of polio cases was down, but the number of health workers on the polio eradication program that were murdered reached eighty over ten years.

Distrust of science: Some people believe that there is wisdom within the body that is far superior to the finite minds of scientists. The measles, mumps, rubella vaccine, known as MMR, is believed by some—in spite of unequivocal evidence to the contrary—to cause autism. The conspiracy theorists believe doctors know the risks but are all in the pockets of Big Pharma, and are trying to line their own, colluding therefore with the government. Donald Trump, the previous president of the United States, has tweeted at least thirty times that he is opposed to vaccination in "one massive dose," and has expressed "no doubt" that they cause autism, and that "the doctors lied."

The truth is that vaccines are not given in one massive dose, and studies on tens of thousands of patients in the UK, Japan, and Denmark, as well as several studies in the US, have failed to show any association between MMR and autism.

Conspiracy theories are enhanced by the internet. They are delusions, the definition of which is "mistaken beliefs that cannot be changed by reason."

There were 41,000 cases of measles in Europe in the first six months of 2018 as a consequence of low vaccination rates. It was the highest rate in ten years. In 2018, the US also suffered several publicized outbreaks of measles associated with refusal to vaccinate.

It is worth repeating: Cotton Mather wrote, *But never any patients had so many pustules of the small pox, as there were lies now daily told and spread among our deluded people.*

John Snow wrote in the 19th century: *We must do away with that form of liberty to which some communities cling, the sacred power to poison to death not only themselves but their neighbours.*

Vaccines, and in particular the smallpox vaccine, have saved millions of lives. Since 1924, 100 million cases of polio, measles, rubella, mumps, hepatitis A, hepatitis B, diphtheria, and pertussis have been prevented. And yet ... people will always worry about safety, will have libertarian fears, and will distrust doctors and drug companies. All of these questions represent reasonable concerns and are to be heard and answered. But with delusional thinking, every evidence against the delusional thought is deemed to be part of the conspiracy. So, the critics will always be with us and the task of public education about vaccines never ends.

Roughly 95 percent of American children receive vaccines as recommended by the medical profession.

POSTSCRIPT

On November 19, 1863, at Gettysburg, Abraham Lincoln delivered a speech in spite of a headache that had been troubling him. He managed to keep it short. As he approached the end, his exhaustion was such that he needed all his resolve to finish. He reached the peroration: "That government of the people, by the people and for the people shall not perish from the Earth."

He slipped coming off the podium, looking "haggard and pale." He was hurried off to the presidential train, and by the time he reached Washington, DC, he had a high fever. Two days later, he developed a diffuse red rash, the "prodrome," and over the next day small, widely scattered blisters covered his body. He was ill for a month. His devoted manservant, William Johnson, developed fever and rash and died. The president continued to work as he could. When told of the crowded anteroom filled with petitioners waiting to talk to him, he joked, "At last I have something I can give everybody."

A bit over a century later, smallpox was eradicated from the face of the earth. The benevolent side of Sitala had won. She had condescended to cure all humans of her disease.

> *Victory! Victory to Sitala Bahrani*
> *Victory, Mother of the Universe, repository of all qualities*
> *You protect the lives of children, O giver of happiness.*
> *Adorned with pure broom and a water vessel in your hand,*
> *The lustre of your forehead is like the Sun.*

> **~from** *Prabhudas, Sitala Calissa*

CHAPTER 11

....

MOSQUITOS IN MEMPHIS: YELLOW FEVER

By 1878, Memphis, Tennessee, had seen multiple epidemics. Four of yellow fever, one of cholera, and some malaria. It is a river port and a crossroads. These are dangerous characteristics for a city to have in a pandemic.

Until 1855, Memphis was thought to be too far north to suffer from these infections, so when New Orleans was scourged by yellow fever that year, Memphis welcomed refugees from the south. This led to the death of three hundred Memphians and with them the myth of immunity. Yellow fever was brought up the Mississippi by riverboat or by railroad. These were the channels of contagion.

Yellow jack, as the disease was commonly known, came to Memphis via New Orleans from Cuba. In Cuba it was known as *enfermo estranjero*, stranger's disease, among other names. The pattern of outbreaks on the island was occasional yearly cases with epidemics every five or ten years of varying severity. The year 1878 was the tenth year of Cuba's War of Independence from Spain, although few in Memphis were paying much attention to that. Yellow fever was severe in Cuba, but war and disease did not prevent trade. Merchant vessels from Boston, New York, Charleston, New Orleans, Rio de Janeiro, Recife, Accra, and Lagos docked beside one another in Havana. Along with their cargo, these ships were bringing the mosquito *Aedes aegypti* from Africa or were taking it to new habitats. When mosquitos eat blood from infected humans, it will be ten to fourteen days before they can squirt virus-positive saliva into the next victim. It will then be four or five days before fever begins. Other mosquitos will then siphon the tainted blood from these patients. This is the cycle of infection. Mosquitos had already adapted easily to the plentiful swamps of New Orleans.

Ships coming into New Orleans harbor were required to serve a fourteen-day quarantine signified by flying a yellow flag known, coincidentally, as the yellow jack. The waiting period was not always followed to the letter. In the case of yellow fever, this laxity with quarantine didn't make the slightest difference. Mosquitos flew off the ships. Infected men, apparently healthy, went ashore.

Memphis, four hundred miles north of St. Louis, was built on bluffs overlooking the Mississippi. It was . . . unhygienic. Sewage festered in the bayou. The *Aedes aegypti* mosquito flourished. Summertime in Memphis is hot and humid, and few Memphians would utter the phrase *It's yellow fever weather*, for fear of tempting Providence. In late July 1878, the mosquitos were unbearable. News came of an outbreak of yellow jack in New Orleans.

Omens were seen. In Memphis, a man was struck by lightning. A five-and-a-half-foot rattlesnake was killed in the city. Strangest of all was the solar eclipse on July 29, just as the first few cases were being diagnosed. The same portent preceded the bubonic plague in Constantinople 1,300 years earlier. And if that weren't enough, there had been a solar eclipse just before the 1793 outbreak of yellow fever in Philadelphia.

CITY PANDEMICS

Plagues in cities follow a pattern little changed since Thucydides described the Plague of Athens in 430 BCE. Don't forget, the cause of the plague was as unknown to the late 19th-century citizens of Memphis as it was to the citizens of Athens before Christ. This is the pattern:

The nearest port declares an epidemic. Despite the denial of danger by the authorities, this leads to flight. Procopius wrote in the 6th century that the best response to pestilence is *Cite Fuego, Vade Longo, Redetarde*—run away quickly, stay a long time, come back slowly. When the news of yellow fever in New Orleans arrived in Memphis, half the population left. By buggy, train, or steamboat, all those who were able found a way to join the refugees already coming from the south. Tables set for dinner were left behind; doors to homes were left wide open. The roads were blocked with traffic. Train ticket prices skyrocketed. People trampled over one another. Near panic swept the city. The population of Memphis in July 1878 was 47,000, and by September it was 19,000. Of those who remained, most lacked the means to leave and 17,000 were to acquire yellow fever.

Some efforts at quarantine were undertaken. People fleeing New Orleans were not permitted to get off the trains in Memphis. A cordon was set up about eight miles around the city, and police with shotguns enforced the line. No one could drive in; no one could get off the riverboats. Elsewhere in the valley, bridges were burned, and train tracks were torn up.

Those who remain sicken and die. A man with fever stayed at the house of the attorney general, G.P.M. Turner. He quickly recovered. Seven days later, Turner's two children complained of fever; one died. In the *Memphis Daily Appeal*, an editorialist wrote, "Yellow Fever rumors have abated . . . this should effectively dispose of the tale circulated by the sensationalists about the presence of Yellow Fever here." This complacency is based on protecting business interests and presages the denialism in San Francisco of the bubonic plague in 1900, Mayor Ed Koch's minimalizing statements about AIDS in 1981, and President Trump's early dismissal of the SARS-CoV-2 pandemic in 2020.

On August 1, William Warren entered a pub, brothel, and gaming den called The Golden Crown, which is not unusual behavior for a deckhand off a riverboat from New Orleans just cleared from quarantine. The next day, he had a headache and a fever. He blamed it on a hangover. He suffered chills, muscle pain, nausea, and vomiting. After four days of infection with yellow jack, many begin to recover. Twenty percent of these will sicken again and go on to develop jaundice and vomit blood. Warren became yellow. Delirium and death followed on day seven.

On August 14, Mrs. Bionda, owner of a snack house, died, leaving her two children and husband behind. Her body was burned within hours and her house and those around were "disinfected" with sulfur fumes, carbolic scrubbings, fire station hosing, and timed explosions to drive the miasmas away. The *Memphis Appeal* editorializes, "The sad case of Mrs. Bionda does not prove necessarily that others will follow. There is no need to panic or stampede." Shortly thereafter, the purgatory begins. Like five hundred cities before it, Memphis becomes a city of corpses.

Forensic pathologists agree that the smell of a rotting corpse is the most pervasively noxious odor. You can't seem to get rid of it no matter how often or thoroughly you shower. The disgusting bleak vileness clings to your nostrils. The stench was everywhere in the streets of Memphis that August. Cologne and rosewater are mixed with the smell, hanging in the air. There are piles of coffins on Main Street. Death wagons often driven by recently freed African Americans are full, or soon to be filled. They actually shout, "Bring out your dead." Houses are burnt. Quicklime is thrown over the corpses lying in the gutters. Fires are made in the streets, fueled by bedclothes, furniture, chamber pots, leftover food—anything "contaminated" by yellow jack. These precautions don't make any difference. The disease is not transmitted by these "fomites."

Social order breaks down. Corpses piled up as early, well-intentioned attempts to bury or cremate the dead declined. First, graves were dug for each individual, then several corpses were put in a shallow grave. Finally, bodies are left to decompose on the street. The smell is overwhelming.

As the tragedy unfolded, compassion waned. The elderly were turned out of doors. People walk down the middle of the street wearing scarves soaked in vinegar or camphor, coughing at smoke from the tar and pitch fires lit to drive the miasmas away. Few people greet one another; no one shakes hands. The healthy were not allowed to touch the dead. The carriers wore gloves.

Victims are found dead in parks, in alleyways, and alone in their deserted houses. Children are found in bed with their dead parents. A starving infant tries to feed from his dead mother's breast. Many die from malnutrition and dehydration. High fever and organ failure lead to delirium. The sufferer is irritable and becomes irrational without any concept of time or place. Hallucinations occur with visions that may be friendly or persecuting. The sick may run down the streets as if possessed. These visions usually precede death.

Bells tolled constantly until the practice was stopped as the constant ringing was bad for morale. This echoed an identical edict in London in 1605 during a bubonic plague outbreak.

There was heroism and villainy. The villains are anonymous: they are looters, thieves, and murderers. The heroes are the saint-like women and men who tend to the sick, risking death themselves. Sister Constance and Sister Thecla worked unceasingly. Their first task was to feed and care for the orphans whose numbers were increasing daily. Next, they must attend to the full to overflowing hospital. It is a dangerous place, so doctors and nurses are few. They don't know the disease is not contagious.

The upper classes chose to be ill at home. The highest mortality was found among German and Irish immigrants. African Americans, freed slaves, were relatively resistant to yellow fever. This had been noticed since the 17th century. If infected, the disease ran a milder course in this population. Anyone who survived yellow fever was immune for life. In earlier years, slaves off the boat might be immune, having been infected in Africa as children. This could not explain immunity found in later generations, which was attributable to an inherited immunity from their forefathers who had lived in endemic areas of West Africa.

The usual self-serving explanations were trotted out. God gave the black man immunity to yellow fever so he could work harder in the fields. White people who did black man's work just brought the disease on themselves. The immune ex-slaves acted with great conscience, working in hospitals and burial teams.

Someone or something that is not the cause of the plague is blamed. Northern newspapers blamed Mardi Gras. "These celebrations of debauchery weakened people's resistance." If so, it was hard to see how Sister Constance, who had been christened thirty-two years earlier as Caroline Louise Darling, complained of a headache after four weeks of tireless work, developed a fever, and died three days later. Sister Thecla got the fever, too, but survived. Many others perished. The nuns who gave their lives are known as the Martyrs of Memphis.

Of 111 doctors who stayed to help the sick, 54 acquired yellow fever and 33 died. This level of service is all the more poignant as none of their treatments had the slightest beneficial effect and often hastened death.

Dr. Mitchell was the physician in charge of the city's response. At first, he asked for help, and volunteer doctors bravely came from as far away as New York. They were particularly likely to die compared to those who had worked in the Mississippi Valley. *Strangers' disease*. Dr. Mitchell eventually asked the volunteers to stay away.

The physicians of the city would meet in the evening at the Peabody Hotel and compare notes. Masks were worn. Some saw between a hundred and a hundred and fifty patients in a day. They used the word *poison*, not disease or infection. A high incidence of miscarriage and stillbirth was noted. Mitchell observed that the disease was not the same as the one he saw in 1873. It was worse.

Two hundred people a day were dying in the city. Sometimes the disease would relapse in an individual and then it was time to "order the coffin"—an acknowledgement of the certainty of death. Most believed that all you had to do was survive until winter. "With the first frost, the epidemic will end." No one knew why.

On September 11, Dr. Will Armstrong, a local practitioner and veteran of earlier epidemics, wrote to his wife, "There is hope that this cool rainy night will possibly end our labors." By September 20, he was dead from the disease.

Famine. Commerce ground to a halt. The city went bankrupt and lost its city charter. Supplies dwindle, hunger follows. Yet there will be no famine in Memphis. There was a national campaign, mostly from northern contributors, to raise and transport millions of dollars in aid, medicine, and food to the southern states. The southerners recognized this aid for what it was, an olive branch and a reincorporation of the South into the postwar nation. It also led to investment in public health infrastructure and the creation of a National Board of Health.

When the epidemic in a city comes to an end, it is forgotten, or more precisely the memory is suppressed. When normality finally returns, political power is weakened. It changes. The empire may fall apart. There is more misplaced blame.

The death toll reached twenty thousand in the Mississippi Valley, and the financial loss was calculated to be $150 million. The toll in Memphis alone was, as Molly Caldwell Crosby pointed out in her book *The American*

Plague, higher than the San Francisco earthquake, the Johnstown flood, and the Great Fire of Chicago combined. *Aedes egypti* had destroyed Memphis. Mortality among whites was 70 percent, and in blacks 8 percent with children under five the most vulnerable group.

The pivotal role of the mosquito in the transmission of the yellow fever virus was completely unsuspected. Yet, if you could have gone back in time to tell them, it wouldn't have made any difference.

THE MOSQUITO AND YELLOW FEVER

Dr. Carlos Juan Finlay of Cuba had been shouting at the top of his lungs about mosquitos since 1872. In 1884, he presented a paper to the Royal Academy of Cuban Medicine entitled *The Mosquito Hypothetically Considered as the Agent of Transmission of Yellow Fever.* He even found the right mosquito—*Aedes,* although it was called *Culex* in those days—and that it was the female that transmitted whatever it was that caused the disease. He ended his paper thus: "It will be with great pleasure that I will listen to any remarks or objections which my distinguished colleagues may deem proper to make."

No one said a word.

The unspoken objections nonetheless hung heavily in the air. *Now come on, Carlos, old boy, obviously yellow jack is caused by failure of temperament, miasmas, fomites, a weakness of personal hygiene, water containing the evacuations of patients with the disease. Obviously! That Italian chap, Sanarelli, he's come up with a bacteria, hasn't he? Very interesting stuff. There are all these Germans and Irish coming into Memphis these days. Now I'm not saying anything, just, you know, you must admit it is a coincidence. And some of the stories I heard about Mardi Gras this year—well, maybe there was a little bit too much of the you know what. The Almighty has His ways.*

Carlos Finlay lived in Cuba through political turmoil. His father was a Scottish physician and planter, a long way from the banks of the Clyde where he was born. His mother was French. His parents met in Trinidad. Finlay was born Cuban and was proud of it, although he was apolitical unlike his three sons who fought for Cuban independence. He studied in

France, but an attack of *chorea* and then typhoid brought him back to the island to recuperate. He finished his medical studies in the United States.

In the 1880s and '90s, the repression of the Cubans was severe. Yet when the United States invaded the island in August 1898, following the sinking of the USS *Maine* in Havana harbor, Dr. Finlay offered his services to the Americans. He had, after all, qualified as a physician at the Jefferson Medical School in Philadelphia. He made his research available to them. The Spanish American War didn't last long. The American army lost four hundred men to Spanish bullets and two thousand to yellow jack.

Second Lieutenant Dr. Walter Reed was made head of the US Army Yellow Fever Commission. It was the third such investigation in Cuba. Finlay was telling anyone who would listen through the first two commissions that the disease was transmitted by MOSQUITOS. He called for mosquito control. Finlay told them, quarantine will not work, burning the fomites (the material contaminated with excrement and vomitus) will not work because, you see, it is transmitted by MOSQUITOS ... At the same time, Reed was busy discrediting *Bacillus icteroides*, a bacterium wrongly thought to be the cause of yellow fever. Dr. Jesse Lazear was second in command of the commission. Their team quarantined and they isolated. They ignored the mosquitos. They put people with malaria and yellow fever together in the same field hospitals. Progress was slow. They knew of Carlos Finlay. They probably exchanged glances when his name came up and discreetly rolled their eyes over his mosquito obsession. No doubt they were committed scientists working hard to solve the vexing riddle of yellow fever. They were operating on what was known at the time about the disease.

1. It was not contagious. An American medical student called Stubbins Ffirth had drunk black vomit—*vomito negro*—in 1804 without ill effect. Without acquiring yellow fever, at least. He rubbed stool, saliva, and vomitus into cuts on his arms, and although they became swollen, he did not get yellow fever. Although aware of his experiments, many could not accept that disgusting fomites were innocent of transmitting the disease. So, his courageous/foolhardy work was not given much credence.

2. The infection varied in severity. The overall mortality was 30 percent. The more African you had in you, the less likely you were to die.

3. It was brought to the Caribbean by slave traders. The first major epidemic recorded in the western hemisphere was on the Yucatan Peninsula in 1648. Over the next two hundred years, there were at least twenty-five major epidemics in the cities of the young United States. First New York, then Philadelphia, then Washington, and then again in Philadelphia. In 1793, 10 percent of the population of Philadelphia died, about four thousand souls.

At last, for want of progress, Reed and Lazear met formally with Carlos Finlay. He gave them some *Aedes* eggs. Reed was deeply skeptical, but he gave the go-ahead to Jesse Lazear to try and infect some volunteers. Reed then had to leave the island on army business. His last words to Lazear were, "Mosquitos are harmless."

Lazear set about his experiments. He isolated a mosquito in a tube stoppered with cotton wool and fed it on a patient with yellow fever. Then he removed the cotton wool and inverted the glass tube on the forearm of a volunteer until the insect fed. He repeated this on twelve people. None became ill.

Ten days later, he came across a tube containing a mosquito that had been fed on the forearm of a patient with yellow fever but hadn't been used in the experiment. Lazear asked his colleague, a Dr. Donald Cooper, if he could use his blood to feed his mosquito. Two days later, Cooper got fever. Using the same mosquito, Lazear let it feed on another volunteer. Ethically and bravely, he inoculated himself along with the volunteer. All three men developed yellow fever. Two survived. Jesse Lazear's wife was at home in the States to deliver their child when she received the telegram. Her husband was dead before she knew that he was ill.

Walter Reed returned to Cuba in a cool fury. The death of his colleague was hard to bear. Of course, he now realizes, it was the mosquito. He is passionate about proving it. He builds two huts. In one, volunteers sleep with filthy fomite-ridden bedclothes from patients with *vomito negro*. In the other he has (paid) volunteers on either side of a grill through which

Aedes cannot pass. On one side there are no mosquitos; on the other side are mosquitos that have fed on infected patients.

Reed also had an insight. Dr. Herbert Carter, part of the commission working with Reed on Cuba, showed him a paper he had written when in Mississippi. He noted an interval of twelve days between the first case in an outbreak and those that follow. Here was an explanation as to why the first twelve people Lazear had initially treated did not get infected. The "germ" has to spend twelve days in the mosquito before it is transmissible.

Reed's experiment showed that only volunteers in the hut with mosquitos that fed on infected patients acquired yellow fever. Within a year, mosquito control interventions eradicated yellow fever from Cuba. Finlay was right.

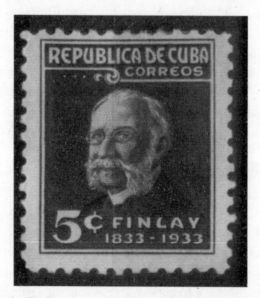

Carlos Finlay memorialized on a Cuban postage stamp.

Yellow fever was the first human disease shown to be caused by a virus, but that discovery did not happen until 1928. Although they made the connection between yellow fever and mosquitos, Walter Reed and his co-discoverers, Carlos Finlay, Jesse Lazear, and Herbert Carter, would not have known of such microorganisms.

Yellow fever is an infection that arose within the last 1,500 years in African primates with transmission to humans by *Aedes egypti*. It is a single-stranded RNA virus typical of those found in the African rain forest, a subject we shall return to. The first known event of this kind, it started in the east of the continent and spread west—it wouldn't be the last.

It is also an unexpected consequence of the slave trade. The disease scourged the Caribbean islands in six or seven epidemics in the 16th century. The circumnavigator and pirate Sir Francis Drake died from it. His death exemplified the risks undertaken by officers and men of the British, French, Spanish, and other navies who also had scurvy and typhus to contend with.

Yellow fever is named for the patient's jaundice, or yellow discoloration seen in the skin and whites of the patient's eyes. Liver failure eventually occurs as the organ cannot synthesize the proteins necessary to clot blood, so such patients have a tendency to bleed. They vomit dark blood, *black vomit*, or *vomito negro*. The disease is also known as the S*affron scourge, Xekic, the American Plague, Fiebre Maligna Putrida, Pestilencias, Matzlahuatt,* and *Cocolitale*, although the last two Aztec names have been applied to measles and smallpox as well. Caribbeans used to call it *Poulicantina*. Some believed it had been imported from Siam. *Mal de Siam.* The Yankees called it yellow jack. It spread to North America. It spread back to Spain. It repeatedly scourged the port cities of the young United States. Through the 17th, 18th, 19th, 20th, and 21st centuries, it has scourged the world.

THE CONTINUING COST OF VIROLOGY

In 1928, Adrian Stokes, a forty-two-year-old family man with two daughters, was head of pathology at Guy's Hospital in London. From a prominent Dublin medical family, he was known for his studies of typhus, cholera, and leptospirosis in the trenches of World War I.

Stokes took a six-month sabbatical to go to Lagos, Nigeria, to study an outbreak of yellow fever. Hideyo Noguchi, a researcher affiliated with the Rockefeller Institute in New York, already famous for showing that neurosyphilis was caused by the spirochete *Treponema pallidum*, was convinced yellow fever was due to a type of bacterium, a spirochete, and overall his views held sway in the medical community.

Stokes worked in the lab in Lagos performing autopsies on monkeys, and during the time he was there, a man from the Hausa tribe named Asibi had a short febrile illness from which he recovered. His illness had the clinical features of yellow fever, so blood was taken from him and injected into a rhesus monkey, number 253A. The monkey developed a febrile illness with jaundice and died. From additional experiments, Stokes was able to show that rhesus monkeys could be infected with blood from infected humans before, and after, passing the blood through a filter that removed all bacteria. In those days, viruses were known as "filter-passing agents." Stokes's experiment demonstrated that yellow fever is caused by a virus and not Noguchi's spirochete, as had been assumed. As Stokes was describing his findings, he realized he had a headache. Lying on what was to be his deathbed, he insisted that uninfected *Aedes aegypti* mosquitos feed on his leg. They did, and they transmitted disease to monkeys. Later, his blood was injected into rhesus monkeys and they acquired yellow fever. Proof! But what a cost. Stokes's paper showing the viral cause of yellow fever was published posthumously. He was buried in the European Cemetery in Lagos. Asibi was given a pension by the Colonial Office.

The viral origin of yellow fever slowly gained acceptance. However, between 1927 and 1931, there were thirty-two reported cases of lab-acquired yellow fever. Noguchi, an erratic genius, was invited by Dr. W. A. Young, a British researcher, to work with him in Accra. Noguchi felt that Stokes's work put his reputation at risk. Young and Noguchi's collaboration was not a happy one as Noguchi's lab habits were ill disciplined. Both he and Dr. Young acquired yellow fever in the Gold Coast and died from it. Before he died, it is said Noguchi acknowledged Stokes's work and conceded the viral origin of yellow fever.

Three years later, Max Theiler, a South African working at the Rockefeller Institute in New York, makes the first effective vaccine using an attenuated version of the Asibi strain. The electron microscope had not yet been invented, so in order to see a photograph of the yellow fever virus, it would take until Doctors G. H. Bergold and J. Weibel showed images in Caracas, Venezuela, in 1962.

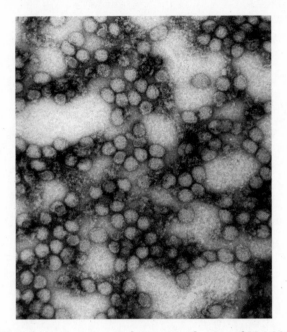

Yellow fever virus seen under a magnification of 234,000×.

The earlier statement that this infection scourged the world is slightly overstated. Some Far Eastern countries, particularly China, appear exempt. Why this should be is not known. Most of these countries have *A aegypti* populations. In fact, the same mosquito also transmits dengue fever, which is endemic in China.

In 2016, ten Chinese people who had been working in Angola in the midst of a yellow fever epidemic flew home from Luanda to Beijing and became the first people reported to have yellow fever in China. Unease surrounds the risk of the infection becoming established there, but so far it has not happened.

In Brazil in 2017, an epidemic of yellow fever began in Minas Gerais and was soon spreading through the country. It is still active.

The disease is very much with us, abetted by an increase in the number and range of mosquitos, a rise in international travel, and an inexplicable worldwide shortage of vaccine.

CHAPTER 12

· ·

THE GREAT DEATH: SPANISH FLU

B revig Mission, Alaska, is north of Nome near the Bering Straits where *Homo sapiens* crossed into North America for the first time 17,000 years ago. It is populated by Inupiat people, about four hundred in number in 1951.

A white-haired man is telling a story.

"In 1918, men brought supplies from Teller by sledge. We helped them unload. Two days later, we are all sick. Coughing with fever and weak. There were eighty of us. Seventy-two died over five days, adults, children, all. The bodies lay on the ground. Of the survivors, I am the only one still living here."

He stops talking.

Listening is Johan Hultin, aged twenty-six. He is an immigrant to the United States from Sweden and has a master's in pathology. He is in Brevig because he wants to exhume the corpses of the victims of the 1918 flu preserved in the permafrost and perform autopsies on them. He is hoping to find virus in the tissues.

The Elders of Brevig have granted him permission.

In the days to come, Johan Hultin will light fires over the mass grave of Brevig and dig. He will repeat the process over and over. It is hard work, but he finds his first corpse after three days. He takes samples of lung from four bodies, then he fills in the graves. After two weeks, he packs his precious cargo in ice bags and thanks the people. The Elders of Brevig watch him climb into a truck and drive off toward Nome.

Fifty years were to pass before Johan Hultin returned. When he did, he wanted to exhume corpses from the mass grave a second time.

SPANISH INFLUENZA

Spanish influenza came in three infamous waves. The first was in March 1918. Unseasonable flu implies, we now know, a new genetic variety of virus. It lasted for four months. The second, most lethal wave spread from early September to the middle of November, scourging the world. The incidence declined only to return in mid-December through April to linger on in isolated communities until the end of that year. No epidemic has ever followed this unusual pattern before or since.

The first wave, active in the Lower Forty-Eight, somehow passed by Alaska. Aware, then, of what might be coming, the governor, Thomas Riggs, put up quarantine in the ports and locked down the schools, churches, theatres, and pool halls. In spite of these efforts, the flu slipped through. In the same way that the infection brought by Columbus on his second journey to Hispaniola in 1493 killed the indigenous people at a rate far in excess of those of European origin, influenza devastated the Inuit.

The grim statistics in Brevig were also found at Teller and Nome. When the villages farther west had not been heard from, miners and their dog teams went to investigate the backcountry. They found frozen bodies huddled together in igloos, some decomposing. Humans ate their sled dogs; dogs fought over human remains. In the Haines area, eight of 150 survived. Many died indirectly. With no ability to feed the fires, they froze to death. Starvation in this subsistence population was widespread. It is estimated that 60 percent of the indigenous people of Alaska died from Spanish influenza or its consequences.

Harold Napoleon is a Yu'pik, which means "real human being." He wrote a book called *Yuuyurak: The Way of the Human Being*. His tribe is closely related to the Inupiat of Brevig and he believes that Alaska's indigenous tribes lost their culture and identity in the Spanish flu. It killed the leaders and the best hunters. It destroyed beliefs and practice. In his language, it is called *yuut tuqurpallratni*, the Great Death. It paved the way for missionaries and teachers and a new way of life to which many could never adapt. Influenza the destroyer.

Influenza, from the Italian for *influence*, meaning influence of the stars. Dis-aster . . . evil from the stars. The influence of the stars causes *catarrh*, from the Greek, a flowing down. Hippocrates (460–370 BCE) described the "Cough of Perinthus," an illness most likely influenza, in his sixth book of *Epidemics*. The word *influenza* has been in use to describe the familiar illness at least since 1510, the year the first pandemic is documented to have spread from Asia through Northern Africa and Europe. It spared the newly colonized Americas somehow. No matter what it has been called, everyone knows "flu." Everyone is familiar with the runny nose, sore throat, fever, headache, and cough. The aches and pains in the joints and muscles accompanied by severe exhaustion leave little option but to take to one's bed.

Flu epidemics have returned again and again. It is seasonal, occurring yearly in the winter. It's a nuisance. It is treated with some respect because very young children, older members of the household, and pregnant women are prone to serious, sometimes lethal, infection. It is not a disaster like the plague; nothing is like the plague, *grazie a Dio*. Each generation forgets the last pandemic and shrugs its shoulders at yearly sporadic flu.

Flu pandemics, an exaggeration of the normal seasonal variety, tend to occur about three times a century. They could have unique features, perhaps nausea and vomiting, conjunctivitis or diarrhea, or higher than usual mortality killing even healthy young people. When that happens, the *previous* epidemic is scrutinized, looking for clues to predict the behavior of the new one, as well as make this and future ones less devastating. Whatever is learned is often forgotten and must be learned anew.

In April 1918, the first reports of what was to become the Mother of All Pandemics came from Spain. Because the country was a noncombatant in the Great War, its press was uncensored. Communications from Madrid told that many, including King Alfonso XIII, had fallen sick of a "strange epidemic disease." From then on, the infection was called the

Spanish Lady or the Spanish flu. The Spanish referred to it as the "Naples Soldier." In the trenches it was known as *Maladie Onze*—Disease Eleven. It had likely been taken to Spain by migrant laborers from France where the disease was raging, abetted by war.

Historians still debate its origin, with three plausible candidates.

1. The army depot at Étaples twenty miles south of Boulogne in France.
2. Camp Funston, at Fort Riley, Kansas; a military depot. Forty-eight doughboys died there in an outbreak of influenza in March 1918.
3. China. In the winter of 1917, Chinese laborers were taken across Canada and the Atlantic to England as much-needed manpower. All along the way, there were outbreaks of the disease.

Whatever the origin, Spanish influenza spread to the four corners of the world. From Alaska to the Pacific islands, from Argentina to Ghana, from London to Los Angeles. It infected one-third of the world's population, killed at least fifty million in just over a year, and then it went away.

Microfiched records from Bellevue Hospital, New York, tell the story. The notes are tragically formulaic: "The patient turned black and ceased to breathe." This phrase is found repeatedly in the clinical notes.

The victims were various: a twenty-four-year-old soldier home on leave, breathless and "heliotrope" blue; a thirty-year-old Irish seamstress; an eight-year-old boy with "mongolism"; an elderly matron of fifty; and a twenty-five-year-old female Polish milliner.

A contemporary approach would be: Give them oxygen! (There was no method for giving oxygen.) Antibiotics! They are dying of secondary bacterial infection! (No antibiotics.) Intravenous fluid! Rehydrate them, at least. (IVs were not generally available.) To the Intensive Care Unit! (But there was no ICU.) The treatment they received consisted of aspirin, morphine, and nursing care. The greatest of these was nursing care. The morphine helped severe breathlessness and it also eased their passing.

At the time, bacteria were beginning to be accepted as a cause of disease. In 1905, Richard Pfeiffer in Germany cultured bacteria from the sputum of half the patients with seasonal flu. Most physicians considered it to be the cause. When the Spanish flu hit New York in 1918, researchers at the Rockefeller University "confirmed" his finding. The bacterium was called *Hemophilus influenzae*, the name it carries to this day. The majority of those who died did so from secondary bacterial pneumonia with bacteria such as *Staphylococcus aureus*, or *Streptococcus pneumonia*, or, yes, *H influenzae* clouding further the search for a causative microbe.

The second cause of death by influenza is the acute respiratory distress syndrome (ARDS). The virus itself targets cells in the alveoli where oxygen diffuses into the bloodstream and carbon dioxide diffuses out. It becomes impossible for oxygen to enter the circulation. The alveoli are blocked by inflammatory cells.

Not everyone at Bellevue Hospital died. The twenty-five-year-old female Polish milliner lingered on. Her fever slowly came down. After ten days, she was discharged back to her family on the Lower East Side.

In the European war zone, in the crowded insanitary trenches, the consequences of influenza were most bitterly felt. Of eleven million military personnel who died, one-third died from disease, of which typhus and influenza were the primary causes. The Germans, in particular, lost heavily to these infections.

The American Expeditionary Force (AEF) were a million strong. In the joke of the time, the doughboys were kneaded, but didn't rise until 1917. During the war, at least 116,708 American soldiers died—over half of them from the flu.

"Black Jack" Pershing, the commander in chief of the AEF, acquired a serious bout of flu a week before the armistice in November 1918. He had suffered from malaria in Cuba when fighting the Spanish but had escaped yellow fever. There were some fears for his life while he was ill. He was in and out of delirium, but after a long illness and a long convalescence, he recovered.

The armistice was set for 11:00 AM Paris Time on 11/11/18. This had been announced two or three days before. Yet the AEF continued to fight and suffered 3,500 casualties on the last day of war from attacking the enemy. A hearing was held in Washington some months later to determine why the decision had been made to attack rather than sit quietly and wait for the armistice. Pershing's answer to the tribunal was that the Supreme Allied Commander, Ferdinand Foch, had not ordered an end to hostilities. Could Pershing's influenza have colored his judgment?

The Spanish flu returned to America with the victorious army, leading to the deaths of a further 675,000 people in the US and lowering life expectancy by twelve years. Celebrations of the armistice were ideal for spreading flu, but by December 18, most parts of the world were free of it. This was the end of the second wave.

Of all the countries of the world, Australia was one of the few that kept the flu out by imposing a strict quarantine. In early 1919, the quarantine was lifted, and then, although it was summertime, the third wave struck, leaving 12,000 Australians dead. Further testimony to the efficacy of quarantine came from American Samoa in the Pacific where the governor, John Payer, insisted it be strictly applied. Not a single person in American Samoa died of flu. In nearby Samoa, an island supervised by New Zealand, ships were allowed to dock and unload cargo, passengers, and crew. Within a few weeks, 8,500 people, a fifth of the population, were dead. Native Americans in South Dakota and indigenous people in the Amazon were at least three times as likely to die of the flu as people of European origin. By May 1919, the epidemic was over except for a last wave of cases in Japan in early 1920.

Viruses were known only to a few in 1918, mostly students of plant diseases. Virology was an obscure, fledgling discipline, and poorly characterized. The medical profession, quite a few members of whom still clung to theories of miasma, was not prepared for creatures smaller than the wavelength of light.

Milton Rosenau, a public health official famous for introducing and sustaining the pasteurization of milk in America, suspected a virus as the cause of the flu and said so. René Dujarric de la Rivière, a French physician and scientist, was convinced that flu had a viral origin. He took blood from four soldiers with influenza, passed it through a Chamberlain filter, which removes all bacteria, and injected it into himself. He got the flu! A week after recovering, he took sputum from another flu patient and painted his throat with it. This did not cause flu and convinced him he had gained immunity from his previous self-induced infection.

Not so fast.

Two other Pasteurians, Charles Nicolle and Charles Lebailly, inoculated a monkey and two human volunteers with filtered sputum, one injected under the skin and the other into the bloodstream. The monkey and the man who received injections under the skin got flu, yet the one who had the concoction injected into the bloodstream did not become ill. It was concluded, correctly as it turned out, that the disease could not be transmitted by blood. How then did Dujarric de la Rivière become sick? He probably acquired it from his close contact with the infected soldiers.

In 1918, an American veterinarian, J. S. Koen, noted that pigs were dying of a very similar disease to that of humans. He thought the cause might be the same in both animals. His views, and indeed the views of all who suspected a virus, were generally discounted.

Yet in 1931, a virus was isolated by Richard Shope and Paul Lewis at the Rockefeller Institute, which caused influenza in pigs, *swine flu*. When it was shown, about this time, that the organism could be transmitted to ferrets, a commonly used laboratory animal, an avalanche of research followed, establishing the science of virology. In 1933, a ferret sneezed into the face of a British scientist called Wilson Smith. He got the flu. Together with Christopher Andrews and Patrick Laidlaw working at the National Institute for Medical Research in the UK, they showed that Shope's virus caused influenza in humans and could be transmitted from humans to ferrets and back again.

THE INFLUENZA VIRUS

The structure of the virus looks simple. It is made of eight strands of RNA in a protein coat. The flu virus is between eighty and a hundred nanometers in diameter and it killed fifty million people.

There are eighteen different hemagglutinin (H) spikes that have been identified so far. They bind the virus to the cells of the mouth and airways. There are eleven neuraminidase (N) spikes. They release the young viruses from the host cell. So, H is the key into the host, and N is the key that lets the virus out of the cell. This mechanism is used to name specific influenza species. H3N9 for instance—H spike 3 binds and N spike 9 releases—causes avian flu. The virus that caused the Spanish flu is H1N1.

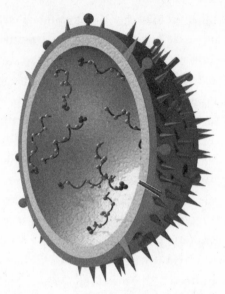

Diagram of an influenza virus. National Institutes of Health.

Flu can be transmitted from an infected to an uninfected person by the former coughing into the face of the latter. It may also travel six feet from a patient simply breathing and talking who is not spitting droplets. You are not necessarily a germaphobe if you believe that you can catch the infection from a bus pole, a doorknob, or a stranger's handshake because the virus can be transmitted by all these means. Once the virus is on your hand and you touch your face then you've made it likely you'll have ten days off from work.

You can also get the virus without touching a surface. The virus wafts into your nose. It enters the cells of the epithelial, or lining, cells in the nose and the airway and progresses down into the lung. While multiplying in those cells, it ultimately destroys them. As the infection subsides, the epithelium heals, a process that can take up to a month, which is the reason cough commonly persists after the acute illness is gone.

The projections on the surface of the virus bind to sialic acid present on the cell surface. It is absorbed into the cytoplasm of the cell, then the RNA is released and translated into protein. This action occurs over and over again. Then the parts of the virus reassemble. One virus goes in, a million come out. It is easy to see that if this process continued unchecked, death would inevitably follow, but thanks to your immune system, it is checked.

Interferons are small proteins from your immune cells. There are many kinds, their actions are subtle, and they are part of the innate immune system. By preventing protein synthesis, they are the first barrier influenza viruses must overcome to enter a cell and multiply. Some have evolved specifically to obstruct influenza. But then influenza has evolved counter-proteins that are antagonistic to interferons. A microscopic arms race is evolving back and forth and has done so over thousands of generations. Unfortunately, excessive activation of the innate immune response leads to massive inflammation that doesn't damage the virus, but the host.

Rubor, calor, dolor, tumor, otherwise known as redness, heat, pain, swelling, are the hallmarks of inflammation. The most virulent viruses induce massive inflammation. In infections such as Spanish influenza and COVID-19, this overreaction of immunity causes more damage than the virus itself. This is the cause of ARDS. It is known as a *cytokine* storm.

HULTIN IN BREVIG, 2

This graph of mortality shows the dotted line, in the shape of a U, which is what you would expect in an influenza epidemic—death in the very old and the very young. The line for the Spanish flu of 1918 is a W. There is a spike of deaths in healthy young people between twenty and forty years of age.

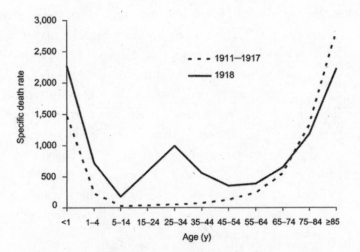

Mortality plotted against age in two influenza epidemics.

In 1997, Hultin is now seventy-two years old and living in retirement on Nob Hill in San Francisco. He continues to ponder the mysteries of the Spanish Lady. He has thought about her intermittently over the last forty years. He hadn't been able to detect virus in the samples he retrieved from Brevig. "It was brilliant work," he would say with a little bitterness, "published in the journal of negative results."

One evening he is leafing through the journal *Science* when he comes across a paper that has him jumping out of his chair. Jeffrey K. Taubenberger and his team at the Armed Forces Institute of Pathology in Washington, DC, have sequenced parts of the Spanish influenza virus from a formalin-fixed, paraffin-embedded lung tissue sample from a soldier who died in the First World War that was kept in the Armed Forces Museum. Nine fragments are sequenced, enough to determine this is influenza A virus H1N1.

Hultin writes Taubenberger a letter with a copy of his CV to prove he is a pathologist and not a lunatic, to let Taubenberger know that Hultin knows where to get better tissue samples. Rather than waiting for the letter to get to Taubenberger, Hultin calls him the next day. Taubenberger's reply is that he will certainly look for virus in any tissue samples Hultin brings to him.

And so, Dr. Johan Hultin, retired pathologist, is on his way back to Brevig, Alaska, on his own dime. In his luggage are a pair of pruning shears that his wife uses for gardening. He flies to Nome and drives to Brevig Mission. It has changed. There is a gas station, a post office, and a mayor. The crosses over the mass grave have gone, knocked over in a storm.

Hultin tells the mayor of his plan to once again dig into the mass grave of those who died from Spanish flu eighty years ago. The mayor has heard of Hultin's first trip and takes his request to the council. The council agrees.

Four young men volunteer to help him with the digging. On the third day of digging, at 3:00 PM, they come upon the first body, six feet down. But the tissue has rotted, which Hultin attributes to the consequences of his digging in 1951. Two feet farther down, he finds the corpse of a well-preserved young woman aged about twenty. He names her Lucy. She is obese, which has protected the lungs. He cuts open her thorax with his wife's pruning shears and removes Lucy's frozen lungs, which are full of blood. He takes tissue from the lungs of three other victims, puts the tissues in preservative, and closes the grave.

Hultin is not worried about catching the virus. "I tried to grow the virus under very good laboratory conditions in 1951 and it was not possible. The virus is dead." By which he means it has lost the power to infect. Before leaving, he replaces the two crosses to commemorate the deaths of the seventy-two out of eighty Inupiat people who died from Spanish influenza at the Brevig Mission in 1918.

The trip has taken him four days. Back in San Francisco (where the mortality of Spanish flu had been greater than in any other US city), he sections Lucy's lungs on the kitchen table and sends them to Dr. Taubenberger by three different carriers.

In less than two weeks, viral RNA is detected in the samples. Dr. Taubenberger proves it has the same H gene he found in the sample from the WWI soldier, and a third pathology specimen shows they all came from the same virus. It takes eight years to complete the RNA sequence. The results are published in *Nature* in 2005.

This *Orthomyxovirus*, this H1N1 negative strand of RNA in eight segments wrapped in protein thirty nanometers in length, killed fifty million people.

The first thing Taubenburger noticed about A/BrevigMission/1/18 (H1N1) was its similarity to the viruses that cause flu in birds. Flu infects creatures ranging from lab mice to lions, but more usually birds, pigs, dogs, cats, horses, bats, whales, ferrets, seals, and humans. But birds are the greatest source. The billions of wild waterfowl and shorebirds of the world are the reservoir for all influenza A subtypes known to exist. Within this reservoir, its genes continually circulate and swap RNA with each other in a process known as reassortment. The virus can spread directly from birds into humans. It can also spread from other animals infected by the birds into humans. Contact with the breath of these intermediate hosts leads to infection. The ability to switch hosts easily is an extraordinary property of the influenza virus. Pigs, for example, are more likely to be infected by humans than vice versa.

By sequencing all collected animal strains, a family tree can be assembled. In 2004, Michael Worobey from the University of Arizona showed that seven of the eight genes in the Spanish flu virus closely resembled flu genes found in birds of North America. The virus jumped from one of these birds to humans a few years before 1918. His research also demonstrates that during the 1872 flu epizootic in horses, the horse virus jumped into poultry and then from poultry to wild birds and from wild birds into humans. This is the likely origin of the Spanish flu, showing it is a North American virus. The first outbreak probably occurred in Kansas.

The reason for its severity can be found in the virus, in the host, and in the bacteria that cause secondary infection. The 1918 virus had a wild waterfowl H1 that led to severe damage to the lining of the human mouth, pharynx, and lung. Healthy humans have an excessive inflammatory response to the virus, and this immune system reaction is so violent that it damages the host more than the virus, producing the now-dreaded cytokine storm. This explains, at least in part, the Spanish flu's predilection for younger people who have a more vigorous immune response. Lastly, this process encourages secondary bacterial superinfection that leads to pneumonia due to strep or staphylococci. Most of those who died of Spanish flu actually died of a secondary bacterial infection.

The flu spreads with remarkable speed. It is a shape-shifting trickster that mutates at a remarkable rate. It escapes from previous immunity by gradually changing the proteins on its coat, known as antigenic drift, by evolving resistance to medicines, and using its astounding evolutionary flexibility. Its ability to mutate is why a new vaccine for seasonal flu is needed every year.

The flu pandemics in the hundred years after 1918, which unfolded in 1957, 1968, and 2009, were all caused by descendants of the virus that caused the Spanish flu. Indeed, the 2009 H1N1 virus was a reactivation of the 1918 H1 gene that had survived for more than ninety years in a pig "time capsule."

So, it is not hyperbole to repeat that the Spanish influenza was the Mother of All Pandemics.

THE SPANISH FLU AND COVID-19

The COVID-19 pandemic began in November 2019 and spread around the world in four months. Spanish influenza spread around the world in a year. Both diseases are acute, feverish, upper respiratory tract infections leading to pneumonia and the adult respiratory distress syndrome, ARDS, with significant mortality. The similarities sparked enormous interest in Spanish flu. This is interesting, as for a hundred years it has been ignored.

The historian Alfred W. Crosby, author of *America's Forgotten Pandemic*, writes about this surprising indifference. After it was gone, it was treated as if it had never happened. *No infection, no war, no famine has ever killed so many in as short a period. And yet it has never inspired awe, not in 1918, and not since.*

In 1924, it was not mentioned in the Encyclopedia Britannica's "most eventful years" of the 20th century. Most contemporary and later histories of World War I omit it or refer to it in passing. It is not in the syllabus of secondary schools that are taught the history of the First World War. Historians woke up to the pandemic around 1968 when "Hong Kong" flu scourged the world. Virologists awoke and reviewed with horror what they had been ignoring. Now, in seeking an understanding of COVID-19, interest in the Spanish flu is higher than it has ever been.

SARS-CoV-2 belongs to a different class of virus than influenza. There are many clinical differences that are covered in Chapter 16. No other virus or other pandemic in history has followed the three-wave pattern of the Spanish flu.

There are practical differences. In 1918, viruses were largely unknown; we can now sequence their RNA or DNA content. A complete sequence of SARS-CoV-2 was available within a month of the plague's onset. Medical care since 1918 has improved with the advent of oxygen therapy, antibiotics for secondary infections, intravenous fluids, and the resources of an Intensive Care Unit, none of which were available at that time. What will happen with COVID-19 cannot be generalized or predicted from the Spanish flu.

Meanwhile, the viruses of the future continue to swirl around us, swapping their genes and evolving in birds, bats, swine, and other animals in an ever-changing pool.

CHAPTER 13

ALWAYS SOMETHING
NEW: HIV

You could think of it as a detective story. There is a sudden rash of unexplained deaths of young gay men in New York City. Dr. Jeffrey Greene, the infectious disease fellow covering Bellevue Hospital on an April evening in 1981, was asked by an intern to see a patient with fever. Dr. Greene examined a pitifully thin twenty-something man who didn't know where he was, couldn't catch his breath, and had thrush on his tongue. The doctor looked at his chest X-ray. Both lung fields were whited out, implying a form of pneumonia.

"We had a similar patient a few days ago," said the intern. "He died."

In hospitals around the city, it was the same story. Doctors quickly came to learn that the same story was playing out across the country, particularly in San Francisco, Miami, and Los Angeles. It was not confined to the United States. In cities across the world, there was an outbreak of this particular pneumonia caused by a fungus, *Pneumocystis*. It was everywhere. At the same time, there was a sudden increase in tuberculosis, brain abscesses, and Kaposi sarcoma, mostly in gay men. For a month or two, the relationship between these disparate epidemics was uncertain. Then it became clear. All of these patients had severely depleted immunity. They had an acquired immune deficiency syndrome.

1896, THE BELGIAN CONGO

Shapes crouched, lay, sat clinging to the earth, half coming out, half effaced within the dim light, in all the attitudes of pain, abandonment and despair.

They were dying slowly—it was very clear. They were not enemies, they were not criminals, they were nothing earthly now—nothing but black shadows of disease and starvation, lying confusedly in the greenish gloom. Brought from all the recesses, fed on unfamiliar food, they sickened, became inefficient, and were then allowed to crawl away and rest. These moribund shapes were free as air—and nearly as thin. I began to distinguish the gleam of eyes under the trees. I saw a face near my hand. Slowly the eyelids rose and the sunken eyes looked up at me, enormous and vacant, a kind of blind, white flicker in the depths of the orbs, which died out slowly.

This passage from *Heart of Darkness* by Joseph Conrad describes the sick men he saw in 1890 near Matadi, the Atlantic port of the Belgian Congo (known today as the Democratic Republic of Congo). The railway was rebuilt in 1920 by African laborers, slaves or near slaves who suffered and died from dysentery, pneumonia, beriberi, and sexually transmitted disease acquired in the prostitution camps. It was in the interest of those building the railway to keep their laboring force healthy. They failed. Between fifteen and thirty thousand out of sixty thousand died.

In 1926, Dr. Pales, the colony's French surgeon, described a new entity he called "Cachexia de Mayombe," translated as "severe wasting or *cachexia* seen in the town of Mayombe." Patients are "an assembly of bones held together by skin . . . whose only sign of life lay in their eyes." He autopsied fifty of those who died. In twenty-six he did not find evidence of a definite medical condition. Some had chronic diarrhea, some had enlarged lymph nodes, and some had shrinkage of the brain, all consistent with AIDS.

When I was working in New York in the 1980s, I would sometimes supervise AIDS patients receiving weeks of intravenous treatment in non-acute wards. They precisely matched Conrad's description. They were, as Dr. Pales described his patients, "an assembly of bones held together by skin."

They wearily pushed their IV poles and leaned on them, gowns flapping. Both Conrad and Dr. Pales accurately described the men I was seeing. The one sign of life, of the human within, was "the bright shining eyes." Had Conrad and Dr. Pales given us the earliest clinical descriptions of AIDS?

The chimpanzee (*Pan troglodytes troglodytes*) lives in the rain forests of Central Africa. It is one of those primates that shares 98 percent of its DNA with *Homo sapiens*. Chimps eat monkeys and they have been infected with simian immunodeficiency virus (SIV) for hundreds of years. The chimp's SIV is a hybrid of simian immunodeficiency viruses infecting two monkeys, the red-capped mangabey and the greater spot-nosed monkey. One particular group of chimpanzees living in Cameroon is infected with SIV chimpanzee virus (SIVcpv), which is indistinguishable from HIV 1 serotype M group B, and causes AIDS in these primates. It spills over into humans. In the rain forest of Cameroon, a hunter, as was common practice, killed a chimpanzee for food—bushmeat. At some point during the killing, skinning, and butchering of one of these apes, the hunter cut himself. The blood of the animal is infectious. Viral transmission from chimps to humans wasn't a onetime occurrence. More than 15 percent of bushmeat handlers are positive for SIV.

Once infected, the patient may stay well for five to fifteen years. Apparently healthy, he or she may transmit the virus through blood, semen, breast milk or vaginal or rectal fluids. Between the years 1985 and 2013, in the US, fifty-eight health care workers, surgeons, nurses, or laboratory workers acquired the infection from cuts contaminated by the infected blood of fellow primates—human patients.

HIV is a prototypical rain forest virus. In technical terms, it is a single-stranded positive-sense RNA retrovirus. This class of viruses has a high mutation rate and is able to move to a new host quickly. There are four groups of HIV—M, N, O, and P. Group M is responsible for the AIDS epidemic. The other serotypes are more common in West Africa and tend to dwindle out locally.

The AIDS virus, HIV 1 serotype M group B, has been in existence since 1908–1920, give or take ten years. Once an HIV-infected man or woman reached large cities like Léopoldville (present-day Kinshasa) or Brazzaville across the Congo Pool, the disease would amplify. We know that the numbers of infected people increased from one or a few cases around 1910 to fifty-five million worldwide in 2007. This exponential growth means that the number of infected people in Kinshasa in 1960 would have been a few thousand and, given the long period of time from infection to disease, it is not surprising that there was little awareness of an AIDS disease at that time.

Because transmission of simian viruses to man had been going on for hundreds of years, the question that must be asked is: What novel factor at the beginning of the 20th century allowed this particular strain to adapt to *Homo sapiens*, leading to a global pandemic of such horrible intensity?

THE SPREAD OF AIDS

On June 30, 1960, Congo became independent from Belgium. Immediately the country fell into civil war. This led to massive shifts of populations to the cities with cultural disruption, expansion of slums and poverty, and the growth of a booming sex industry. In 1960, the capital of the Republic of the Congo, Kinshasa (formerly Léopoldville), had a population of 358,000. In 2020, it is 14,342,000. There are more French speakers in this capital today than in Paris. As we've emphasized elsewhere in this book, the megalopolis is the augmenter of plagues.

But how did HIV get to Kinshasa? It is six hundred miles from Cameroon. The idea of a lonely hunter making his way down the Sangha River into the Congo and then to the capital city where he spreads the infection is plausible but not robust. We need to look at other circumstances that allowed subtype M to thrive and not peter out like other HIV/AIDS-related subtypes.

There is something else, taken together with the social ills of the boomtown, alongside colonialism and post-colonialism, that explains more fully the early spread and establishment of HIV infection.

It is dirty needles.

AIDS was the third new calamitous epidemic the continent of Africa had suffered over a hundred years. As it turned out, the first two led to the third.

RINDERPEST, CATTLE PLAGUE

Italian colonizers imported cattle infected with cattle plague, rinderpest, into Eritrea on the Horn of Africa. From 1888 to 1897, this viral infection devastated the continent from north to south and from east to west. Within five years, it reached the Atlantic, and within ten it had crossed the Limpopo into southern Africa. Mortality in cattle was 90 percent. The virus did not directly infect humans, but people died from the widespread famine that followed. An estimated one-third of the human population of Eritrea died from famine and war, a slaughter from which the country has never recovered. Two-thirds of the Masai people of East Africa died. A Masai elder described how the corpses of cattle and people were "so many and so close together that the vultures had forgotten how to fly." Cholera and typhus exacerbated the famine.

HUMAN AFRICAN TRYPANOSOMIASIS

Famine and war led to ecological change that allowed the tsetse fly to flourish in abundance. The tsetse fly injects the protozoa that causes sleeping sickness, also known as Human African Trypanosomiasis, or HAT, into humans. This was the *second* plague. From 1896 to 1906, it killed half a million people in the Congo. It has been called Africa's Black Death. Without curative treatment, which was limited in the early days, it has a 100 percent mortality.

This epidemic in the Congo led to social and economic upheaval. Africans were being used as soldiers and as laborers for construction projects to harvest rubber and to mine. The death toll was increasing, and the colonial overlords became concerned. Business versus pandemic. You can imagine them thinking: *Who is going to build the roads and railways? Who is going to work in the mines of Katanga, which has 34 percent of the world's cobalt reserves and 10 percent of the world's copper? And how shall we avoid risk to ourselves?*

This is a reprise of the Spanish colonizers' response to the disappearance of the Taino in Hispaniola, and of the Europeans to the demise of the

"Indians" on the continent of North America. In America, the Europeans solved their problem by importing African slaves to do the work. In the Congo, the Belgians had to find a different solution.

The solution to the problem of the natives, or "nos negres" as they were commonly known to the Belgians, was to recruit scientists.

MÉDECIN-COLONEL EUGÈNE JAMOT AND DIRTY NEEDLES

Doctor Jamot graduated from Montpelier University in France in 1909, traveled to Cameroon, and saw firsthand the towns that had been emptied and rendered extinct from the scourge of trypanosomiasis.

His solution was to train teams to go into villages and palpate the necks of the villagers. If they had swollen lymph nodes, the earliest sign of trypanosomiasis, these would be aspirated for microscopic examination.

Needle one.

If the examination under the microscope showed trypanosomes, the team would perform a spinal tap.

Needle two.

If positive, the team would treat the patient with intramuscular atoxyl, or intravenous tryparsamide.

Needle three.

This process became known as the Jamot doctrine. He applied it with great efficiency, visiting and revisiting villages. Within eighteen months, ninety thousand people had been examined and five thousand cases of HAT were identified and treated. He conducted his treatment by using only three microscopes and six syringes. This effort was a huge success against HAT, and his doctrine was repeated and applied to this and other infections, such as yaws and malaria, over the first six decades of the 20th century in Africa.

Unsterile needles continued to be used at a high rate in the Congo. They were found in applying the Jamot doctrine, in STD clinics, in administering medicines, and in vaccination programs until disposable plastic syringes became available. But that was a long time coming: Disposable plastic syringes were not widely available until the early seventies in Europe and North America, later in the Congo.

THE FIVE AITCHES

In the early 1990s, I was in New York City working with AIDS patients at Bellevue Hospital. My colleagues and I found it hard to get away from the subject and found ourselves eating, drinking, sleeping, talking, and dreaming about AIDS. Sixty percent of patients in our hospital were positive for the virus. By then we all knew the risks of dirty needles.

One evening at the Rockefeller University, I met William Ball, a man just back from Cameroon in West Africa. He was a working scientist and he told me about research on the virus HIV2 that showed it existed first in the sooty mangabey monkey. It jumps into humans in the same way HIV1 jumps from chimps into humans and causes a milder form of the disease.

I told him about the "five aitches" that represented the people who are at risk for HIV infection: homosexuals, hookers, heroin addicts, hemophiliacs, and Haitians.

"Haitians? Why Haitians?"

"That's everyone's first question. There are a number of mistaken and prejudicial hypotheses. Some say they are more promiscuous than everyone else."

"Ridiculous."

"Second, now that the virus-out-of-Africa is gaining credibility . . . it turns out that the United Nations peacekeeping force that was sent during the Congo Civil War in the 1960s contained some Haitians. So, they must have caught it and brought it back. There were also Irish, Swedes, and Canadians, of course. And if you don't like that, there is an enormous amount of trade between Haiti and Africa."

"Really?"

"No. There's no trade with Africa. Africa is three thousand miles away. Haiti trades first with the Dominican Republic and then the US. Next door."

"So, why were Haitians on that list of aitches?"

"As many as forty-five hundred Haitians came to Kinshasa in the sixties to run the civil service and the professions, posts filled hitherto, by policy, only with Belgians, who had gone home following independence. The Haitians spoke French, were well educated, and by coming to Africa may have felt some relief from the oppression of living in Papa Doc's Haiti.

"One of them—it could have been just one infected man—brought HIV 1 group M, subtype B back to Haiti in or about 1966. This slightly unusual type was spread into the community so that, by 1982, 8 percent of women attending an antenatal clinic in Port-au-Prince were infected with the virus.

"There were two routes HIV took from Haiti to the US mainland. The first was a consequence of sexual tourism. In the sixties and seventies, gay men, primarily, came from the US to Port-au-Prince looking for sex and paying for it. The association between poverty and prostitution is well understood. At residences such as the Habitation Leclerc and Pension Tropicale, their wishes were catered to. The sex trade didn't contribute a lot to AIDS in Haiti, although it did a little. More importantly, these men got infected and took it home with them."

In Haitian voodoo, Baron Samedi is a spirit noted for disruption, obscenity, debauchery, tobacco, and rum. Which is why everyone loves him, particularly on weekends. He is reminiscent of James Bond—except that he is bisexual. After a brief meeting with Le Baron, tourists would get the infection and go back to New York, San Francisco, or Miami. Within three months to a year of acquiring the HIV infection, patients frequently develop an acute flu-like illness called the acute seroconversion syndrome. While the illness is generally mild, the sufferer is highly contagious.

The second route was selling plasma. The *New York Times* reported on January 28, 1972, under the headline "Impoverished Haitians Sell Blood for Use in the US," that five to six thousand liters of plasma were being sold to the US every month because of local shortages. The company handling the collection and transport of the blood was Hemo Caribbean and it was owned by a Miami businessman. However, the true control of the company was in the hands of Luckner Cambronne, Haitian president Papa

Doc Duvalier's right-hand man. It was literally money for blood. His business only operated for one year, but that was enough. Similar disasters of spreading infection via blood transfusions were to follow in India, Mexico, Spain, and, worst of all, China, where, in one distribution episode, 250,000 people were infected by tainted blood.

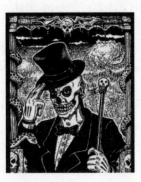

A loa or god of Haitian voodoo, Baron Samedi.

THE AIDS EPIDEMIC

On April 24, 1980, Ken Horne was the first case of AIDS diagnosed in the US.

In January 1983 in Riyadh, Saudi Arabia, a Bedouin camel herder is puzzling his doctors. He has pneumocystis pneumonia. Some word of the disease AIDS has reached the country. Could he have what some call the "gay plague"? Homosexuality is punishable by death in the Desert Kingdom. Blood that had been sent abroad for testing comes back after ten days, positive for HIV. The man has a scar on his abdomen, and questions to his family reveal what happened. Five years earlier, he had been hit by a truck and had been transfused with four units of blood imported from Miami.

In the May 20, 1983, issue of *Science*, the article "Isolation of a Retrovirus from a Patient at Risk for Acquired Immune Deficiency Syndrome (AIDS)" is published. Francoise Barré-Sinoussi and Luc Montagnier identify the virus that causes AIDS. Some years later, they are awarded the Nobel Prize for this discovery.

Thirteen long years are to pass before a treatment is found.

In 1996, Alex S. has one foot in the grave. As his doctor, I think more like one foot and a half. Alex is as thin as a stick, with swollen lymph nodes all around his neck. He complains in a low, defeated mumble of his persisting diarrhea. "I have some new treatment for you," I tell him. He doesn't muster much enthusiasm. His pessimism isn't unfounded. We had seen false hope before with this disease. But at that moment, I hadn't anything else to try.

"It's a bit arduous," I tell him. "It's about thirty pills. You have to take some with meals and some between meals. And some with grapefruit juice. We'll write it out for you."

A week later, Alex is still alive. A month later, his diarrhea has improved. Three months later, the swelling in his lymph nodes has disappeared and he is actually putting on weight. Six months later, he goes back to work as a trainer in a gym. The medicine he takes is called highly active antiretroviral therapy, or HAART. It is not a cure. You must take it for life. But by 2020, one pill a day is all that is needed.

In 2020 in the world:

35 million people have died from AIDS
1.87 million people were newly infected in 2020
1.6 million of these are over fifteen
37.9 million people live with AIDS
23.2 million have access to antiretroviral treatment

Vaccine research continues. Post-exposure prophylaxis, PEP, is a short course of antiretrovirals that can prevent infection with HIV but should only be used in emergency situations.

Human immunodeficiency virus spilled over from chimps to humans in Cameroon. Humans carried it to Kinshasa. From there it diffused through Africa. Sporadic cases spread around the world. It reached the US via Haiti. It spread to all the countries of the world. No one is immune.

This *is* the global era of plagues.

CHAPTER 14

WE WENT INTO THE RAIN
FOREST AND PANDEMICS
CAME OUT: WEST NILE
VIRUS, ZIKA, AND EBOLA

The rain forests of the world are spread around the equator. There are more living organisms and more diversity of living organisms in them than anywhere else on land. They cover 2 percent of the earth's surface (although they are shrinking) yet contain over 50 percent of its flora and fauna. Only the oceans teem with greater biodiversity. Wherever you have life, you have viruses. The more life, the more viruses.

Primates, which include lemurs, lorises, tarsiers, monkeys, chimpanzees, apes, and humans, have the third-highest numbers of species after rodents and bats. All three families are present in huge numbers on the planet. Precisely when modern *Homo sapiens* evolved as an independent primate remains an anthropological puzzle, at least for now. Human remains found at Jebel Irhoud in Morocco dating from three hundred thousand years ago are accepted by most as the earliest example of our species. What no one doubts is that we originated in Africa, leaving the continent approximately fifty to seventy thousand years ago to migrate around the world.

In our African days, we were never far from the rain forests. Early *H sapiens* would have traversed them, looking for food. Contemporary *H sapiens* still does. Bushmeat consists of non-domesticated mammals including pouched rat, duikers, porcupine, chimpanzee, monkey, and gorilla; reptiles, snakes, amphibians, birds—in other words, anything you can eat.

171

Bushmeat is big business. Once limited to rural communities that relied on the meat for subsistence, it has grown into a multimillion-dollar industry to feed an exploding population. In urban Africa it is considered luxury food, and it is even exported, illegally, to cities such as London, New York, and Toronto.

Non-African commercial interests seeking natural resources also penetrate the rain forests looking for minerals or logging, which then leaves open land to graze cattle and raise them for meat. These two forces work together. Roads make it easier for bushmeat hunters to penetrate the forests and to transport their food.

The viruses of the rain forests are not new; they are simply newly discovered. The rodents and the bats that live there are the main reservoirs for viruses. Primates, including us, become intermediate hosts. The viruses have been disturbed in their *sylvatic*, or forest, habitats by *H sapiens* and then they spill over. They are often transmitted by blood-eating mosquitos, lice, and ticks. As global temperatures rise, the number of such insect vectors will also increase.

Humans are useful hosts for viruses because we live in villages, towns, and cities in close proximity to the forests and leave an abundance of standing water in which the mosquito can reproduce. From these areas, the viruses travel in their hosts by trains, boats, and planes around the world.

The inescapable consequence of destroying the rain forest is more plagues.

CROWS FELL TO THE GROUND: WEST NILE VIRUS

July 1999. Dead crows are dropping from the sky onto the pavement of New York in the boroughs of Queens and the Bronx. *Corvus brachyrynchos* had been crashing onto windscreens and thudding to the ground since June. Dead birds falling from the sky has been seen by many cultures as omens of the gods' displeasure. In Queens, it's just a pain, already.

By August, veterinarian Dr. Tracey McNamara, working at the Bronx Zoo, reported, "It's raining crows. Some of them are still alive, just. They can't fly, they shake, they can't balance. It's neurologic." She performed necropsies that showed bleeding in their brains, and under the microscope severe brain inflammation. Shortly thereafter, birds in the zoo began to die unexpectedly. First a bald eagle, then a snowy owl, some flamingos, and then some cormorants. Dr. McNamara called the Centers for Disease Control and Prevention and was told, "We don't do flamingos."

At the Flushing Hospital Medical Center in Queens, forty-eight minutes away by bus from the zoo, two elderly men were dying of encephalitis, or inflammation of the brain. They have the same disease as the crows. Dr. Deborah Asnis, an infectious disease specialist, called the New York Department of Health and the CDC. By the end of this outbreak, eight local people would die from this infection.

Now the CDC was interested. They listened to Dr. McNamara. Pathologists performed autopsies on the dead men. At first, they thought death was caused by St. Louis encephalitis virus. After careful review, it became clear that the infecting agent was the West Nile virus (WNV). This was a big surprise *as it had never been seen in the western hemisphere before.*

WNV is a virus that circulates in birds and mosquitos. *Homo sapiens* and other mammals are dead-end hosts, which means the virus cannot be transmitted from us to others. The mosquito *Culex pippens,* found all over the world, is the primary carrier, although forty-three other mosquito species transmit it as well. Birds can become infected by drinking water in which there are virus-carrying mosquitos. Predator birds may get sickened from eating infected birds.

That winter of 1999, WNV survived in mosquitos in underground sewers and abandoned buildings. The following spring, more birds were infected. Outbreaks occurred along avian migratory routes.

In four years, WNV spread to every state in the union except Alaska and Hawaii. It infected 208 species of bird and 29 species of mammal including skunks, cats, and dogs. It caused severe disease and death in horses. The dead included a lizard, an alligator, and 40 humans. In 2019, the cumulative human death toll total from the WNV epidemic now stands at 2,000 cases reported in the United States. Seven Canadian provinces were also afflicted. In this same period, WNV has been identified for the first time in most Caribbean islands, Meso-America, Mexico, and parts of South America.

Israel has suffered from WNV for many years. When the virus in Queens had its RNA sequenced and compared to a number of viruses around the world, it was identical to the Israeli one. This suggests its origin. It entered the US via an infected man, bird, or mosquito from Israel—there is no evidence to suggest which.

IN THE ZIIKA FOREST

In 1975, two miles along the road from Entebbe airport to Kampala, the capital of Uganda, there was a large broken-down three-story colonial building. A few children played on a neglected, overgrown veranda, as a grandma crouched over an open fire on the front lawn, cooking. A little farther along stood a roadside sign, announcing a research institute in the Ziika Forest.

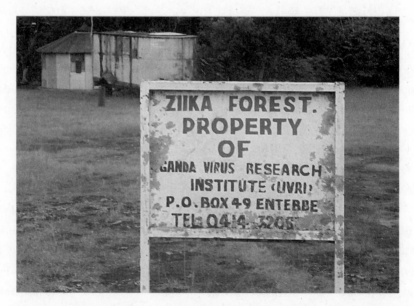

Uganda Research Institute in the Ziika Forest on the shores of Lake Victoria.

Few visitors would suspect that, in that deserted facility, a revolution in virology had taken place. West Nile virus was discovered here. In 1937, a paper in the *American Journal of Tropical Medicine* titled "A Neurotropic Virus Isolated from the Blood of a Native of Uganda" and authored by K. C. Smithburne, T. P. Hughes, A. W. Burke, and J. H. Paul was published. The date of the article is interesting because by then some sixty viruses or "filter-passing agents," as they were also known, had been identified to science. Some of these viruses infected plants, some infected animals, and a handful were known to cause disease in humans, including yellow fever. While looking for yellow fever, the scientists found new antibodies in a feverish young woman in Uganda's West Nile province. This implied a new virus, which they named West Nile.

From 1937 to 1967, in this facility in Uganda, medical pioneers isolated nine human disease–causing viruses. In addition to West Nile virus, they identified, in no particular order:

> *Chikungunya* ("to become contorted" in the Makonde language)
> *Semliki Forest virus*
> *Mengo virus*
> *Ntaya virus*
> *Uganda S virus*
> *Bwamba virus*
> *O'nyong-nyong* (meaning "joint breaker" in the language of the
>   Acholi tribe from Northern Uganda)
> *Kadam virus*
> Zika (The word *ziika*, pronounced *zee eeka*, means "untended
>   forest" in Luganda, the local language)

"Zika Virus. I. Isolations and Serological Specificity" by G. W. Dick, S. F. Kitchen, and A. J. Haddow is a journal article from 1952 in *Transactions of the Royal Society of Tropical Medicine and Hygiene*. Note that an *i* in the name *Ziika* has been dropped along the way. The medical researchers discovered the virus in a rhesus monkey in 1947. The virus could not have been more appropriately named. The stretch of forest along the shores of

Lake Victoria was called Ziika, but the word can mean all forests, which in equatorial Africa would mean rain forest.

Zika virus slowly wended its way toward the Americas in an easterly direction. It traveled from French Polynesia to Brazil, where it exploded around the time of major sporting events like Sprint World canoe racing, the FIFA World Cup, and the Summer Olympics of 2016. The disease spread through South America and into the United States in that year.

Zika virus causes a three-to-five-day fever with a rash. If it's acquired in pregnancy, however, it can lead to babies being born with small heads or no heads at all—called anencephaly. Other viruses, such as rubella and cytomegalovirus, can result in a similar catastrophe.

Currently, eighty-seven countries have *autochthonous*, or indigenous, mosquito-borne Zika. The yellow fever virus that scourged Memphis in 1878 came from the African rain forest. It traveled along with the mosquito and was spread by the slave trade. Dengue fever, also a mosquito-borne illness, came next. The WHO estimates that in 2019 there were 390 million dengue virus infections in 128 countries, 96 million of which had symptomatic illness, and a million died. This is a substantial increase from 2018. You can be infected four times with this virus, also known as "breakbone" fever. In 1789 in Philadelphia, physician Benjamin Rush described an outbreak of what was thought to be dengue fever. From the historical record, you can't tell for sure whether it was chikungunya virus infection or dengue, so similar are their clinical features.

Chikungunya was first described in *Transactions of the Royal Society of Tropical Medicine and Hygiene* in: "An epidemic of virus disease in Southern Province, Tanganykia Territory, in 1952-53. I. Clinical Features," by M. C. Robinson and W. H. R. Lumsden.

Who were these virus hunters? K.C. Smithburne, T.P. Hughes, A. W. Burke, J. H. Paul, G. W. Dick, S. F. Kitchen, A. J. Haddow, M. C. Robinson, and W. H. R. Lumsden made their discoveries without DNA technology and without an electron microscope. They measured antibodies in the blood after injecting mice, monkeys, and hedgehogs with viruses. They were professional medical scientists from the United Kingdom and the US. Their amazing discoveries make them unsung heroes.

EBOLA

Mosquitos are not the only way some rain forest viruses spread to humans. AIDS and hepatitis C virus are RNA viruses from the rain forest that infected non-human primates before they spilled over into us to travel around the world. Another typical rain forest virus, Ebola, whose name means "Black River," has been in the Congo Basin for at least a thousand years. It belongs to the RNA virus species filovirus with an unusual crook in its tail.

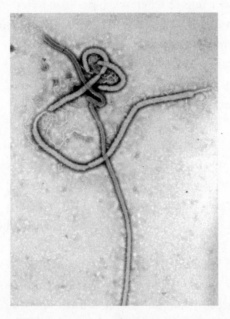

Ebola virus under electron microscopy.
Dr. Frederick Murphy, CDC.

Forest clearing and the bushmeat business allowed Ebola to infect *Homo sapiens*. Its primary host is the fruit bat with occasional spillovers to humans, primates, and possibly other mammals. So, make a note: Never, ever handle bushmeat without gloves, and particularly, do not handle dead bats.

Of the five strains known so far, *Ebola Zaire* has the highest mortality. The death rate is a brutal 90 percent. The biggest epidemic to date was in 2013–16 in Liberia and neighboring countries when 4,809 people died. At that time, eleven people were sick with Ebola in the United States. Two died after having imported the disease from Liberia. The other nine survived and are doing well, which is good news as long-term complications can include arthritis, uveitis, hearing loss, and psychiatric complications.

The second-biggest Ebola epidemic took place in the eastern province of Kivu in the Democratic Republic of the Congo in 2019, with cases in the provincial capital, Goma, on the shores of Lake Kivu. About two thousand have died so far, and relief efforts have been hampered by civil turmoil between rebel groups. The good news is that there may be an effective treatment. Infusions of antibodies, *monoclonal* antibodies, tested in a field trial, have reduced mortality to less than 10 percent. This is exceptionally encouraging and the results of further trials are awaited. More good news: As of 2020, a promising vaccine is currently in trials.

One survivor of the Liberian outbreak, Orphelia, has described how, after losing her husband and son to Ebola, she was blamed for the disease, not allowed to use the village pump, and told, "You killed your husband and son." Anyone who helped her was ostracized. Many continue to believe the disease is caused by witchcraft or conspiracies, one theory of which asserts that international aid services brought the virus with them as part of an unspecified plot.

The best management of Ebola outbreaks includes secure isolation, dignified but safe burial procedures, health education and community engagement, and coordination among health agencies. Optimum effectiveness arises when traditional healers are involved. For all this to happen, it would help to have the absence of war, a competent government, and the abolition of delusional thinking.

———————

Pause for thought.

These viruses identified at the Uganda Virus Research Institute were the beginning of a process of discovery. The increasing numbers of viruses coming out of the rain forest and infecting us is a direct consequence of our intrusion into it.

PREDICT-2 for pandemic prevention was a United States Agency for International Development (USAID) Emerging Pandemics Threat program that for a decade had supported virological, ecological, and epidemiological research around the world. Inspired by doctors at the Uganda Virus Research Institute, PREDICT-2 discovered a thousand novel viruses over an eight-year period. It was closed down a few weeks before the onset of the SARS-CoV-2 global pandemic began.

The Global Virome Project is a ten-year partnership with many countries to build a global atlas of *zoonotic* viruses in their environmental context. This undertaking is under the primary supervision of the World Health Organization. It has been both criticized and applauded. But the effort acknowledges the risk of future plagues and is tackling the problem on an international level.

If we do not learn, the next plague will be a disease never previously thought of. An apt name for it would be the Continuing Revenge of the Rain Forest Virus.

CHAPTER 15

SEVERE ACUTE RESPIRATORY SYNDROME CORONAVIRUS 2 (SARS-CoV-2)

I n a review called "Origin and Evolution of Pathogenic Coronaviruses," published on December 10, 2018, in the American journal *Nature Reviews of Microbiology*, scientists Cui Jie, Li Fang, and Shi Zhengli from the Wuhan Institute of Virology, Hubei, China, warned, specifically, that a global coronavirus pandemic was coming.

Exactly one year later, in 2019, the first human cases of infection with SARS-CoV-2 appeared *in* Wuhan. By January 2021, it had spread to almost all the countries in the world, infecting 100 million and leading to the deaths of 2.3 million with no sign of slowing down.

It originated in bats.

WHAT IS A CORONAVIRUS?

Coronaviruses have the largest RNA genomes known. When RNA replicates, it does so imperfectly. These frequent mutations allow rapid evolution, up to a million times the speed of their hosts. This explains how well such viruses adapt to living in new species and the survival advantage that goes along with it. There are seven coronaviruses that infect people. Four cause the common cold.

On Salisbury Plain in the southwest of England from 1945 to 1989 was a collection of huts called the Harvard Hospital, also known as the Common Cold Unit. It was established for virological and epidemiological research. Twenty thousand volunteers passed through it. There was food, accommodation, and pocket money. Many came back year after year. As a result of the research conducted there, more than a hundred viruses were identified that cause the runny nose, malaise, sore throat, headache, and fever familiar to everyone who has ever had a cold—*the one thing the medical profession can't cure.* Among their number were four coronaviruses known prosaically as 229E, NL63, OC43, and HKU1.

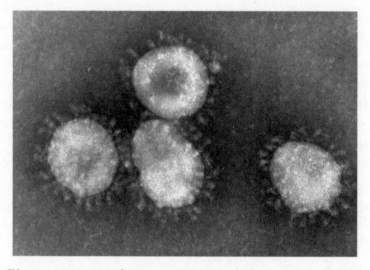

Electron microscopy of a coronavirus, named after its crown of spikes. Latin, corona, *meaning "crown." Dr. Fred Murphy, CDC.*

SEVERE ACUTE RESPIRATORY SYNDROME CORONAVIRUS 1 (SARS-CoV-1)

SARS-CoV-1 is the fifth coronavirus known to cause disease in humans. It came and it went. It caused an outbreak of respiratory disease in Guangdong province in China in 2003 and 2004, spreading to twenty-nine countries, infecting eight thousand people, and killing 774. Eight people in the United States were known to have been infected, none of whom died. Since 2004, there have been no further reported cases. Its origin was the horseshoe bat, which is found in many countries of the world.

It is this virus, SARS-CoV-1, that Shi Zhengli, the senior author of the review referenced above, discovered, isolated, and sequenced. She was known as "the Bat Lady," as she had discovered hundreds of coronaviruses of astonishing genetic diversity in bats in caves across China. It was on the basis of her work with SARS-CoV-1 that she predicted the current pandemic. When SARS-CoV-2 fulfilled her prophesy, she said, "It was Nature punishing the uncivilized habits and customs of humans."

She pointed out that direct infection from bats was rare. These RNA viruses adapt rapidly to different animal species, causing many a pandemic among them. It is the spillover from these intermediary hosts to humans that spreads the virus. Once in humans, transmission from person to person occurs and the pandemic takes off. In SARS-CoV-1, the intermediate host was the civet cat. There were outbreaks in restaurants where palm civets were prepared and eaten. The domestic cat was among the many other animals that were infected.

The virus has much in common with SARS-CoV-2. It enters the cell through the same receptor, known as the angiotensin converting enzyme 2 receptor (ACE2), and it causes a similar disease. It had a higher mortality of 10 percent but was less contagious and soon came under control as a result. It has currently disappeared.

MIDDLE EAST RESPIRATORY SYNDROME CORONAVIRUS (MERS-CoV)

In 2012, the first patient discovered to be infected with MERS-CoV came to a private Saudi Arabian hospital with pneumonia and renal failure and soon died. Dr. Mohammed Zaki, an Egyptian virologist, identified the cause: a novel coronavirus—the sixth coronavirus that causes human disease. The disease resembles SARS-CoV-1 and 2 by causing respiratory symptoms and pneumonia. Diarrhea may be prominent, and the mortality rate of 35 percent is the highest known in coronavirus infections. MERS-CoV is transmitted to humans from dromedary camels. Human-to-human transmission occurs rarely—it does not have the contagious ease of SARS-CoV-2. Twenty-seven countries have reported cases of MERS since 2012, and 858 deaths have been reported as of December 2020.

The seventh coronavirus known to cause disease in humans is SARS-CoV-2.

SARS-COV-2:
THE FIRST INTERNET PANDEMIC

On December 31, 2019, a cluster of pneumonia cases, including seven severe instances that had occurred over the previous three weeks, were reported in Hubei province. Most were connected to the Wuhan Huanan Seafood Wholesale Fish and Live Animal Market, which was closed the next day.

Professor Zhang Yongzhen, a virologist at Fudan University, Shanghai, received a test tube packed in dry ice at 1:30 PM on January 3, 2020. It contained material washed from the bronchial tree of a patient with pneumonia who was on a ventilator in an ICU in Wuhan. Dr. Yongzhen and his team worked nonstop, and forty hours later they had identified the virus and sequenced its RNA genome. It was a coronavirus with 75 percent similarity to SARS-CoV-1. Yongzhen uploaded his sequenced genome to the US National Center for Biotechnology Information on January 5. For emphasis, it was also posted by January 11 on virological.org.

So it was that three weeks after the first reports of COVID-19, the pathogen responsible was identified and characterized. This remarkable event is a milestone in the history of medicine. For example, the virus that caused the Spanish flu that occurred a hundred years earlier was identified eleven years after that pandemic had ended.

SARS-CoV-2, the cause of the disease COVID-19, became the first internet pandemic. Anything that happened anywhere in the world was quickly accessible anywhere else in the world. And with the internet came many COVID-19 conspiracy theories. A popular idea was that the virus was deliberately manufactured, or that it was purposefully leaked from a lab, or it is spread by 5G for some ulterior motive. All these theories have been meticulously and systematically disproven. Not that facts will have any influence on the deluded.

COVID-19 VACCINES

On December 2, 2020, the British government authorized the use of the Pfizer and BioNTech vaccine one year after the onset of the pandemic. If all goes according to plan, it will be 95 percent effective. Of 42,000 volunteers, half of whom were given the vaccine and half given a placebo, 170 acquired COVID-19. Of these, 8 were in the vaccinated group and the other 162 had received placebo.

Let's take a closer look at the mechanism of the action of the vaccine. From Edward Jenner on, vaccines consisted of protein in one form or another from the infection-causing pathogen or one like it that could induce the body to make antibodies that would protect it from the disease.

The Pfizer/BioNTech vaccine introduces strands of synthetic messenger RNA held in lipid particles into our cells. This RNA codes for spike proteins, which stimulates an adaptive immune response against the virus. These antibodies will block it from entering the cell. The primary difficulty with this revolutionary approach is the fragility of the RNA molecule, which rapidly degrades if not stored at −94 degrees F.

A second vaccine has been approved in the USA and in Europe. Manufactured by the pharmaceutical company Moderna, it is also an mRNA vaccine but can be stored at normal refrigerator temperatures.

Unpredicted side effects of the vaccine are possible in spite of studies undertaken to date. At the moment, a painful arm is the dominant complication. Patients with some specific allergies are at risk of severe allergy and should not take the vaccine.

Vaccine Attitudes

A vaccine is a remarkable weapon for humans in the fight against lethal infections, and the discovery and manufacture of effective vaccines within a year of the onset of the pandemic is another example of the primacy of science in this fight. Yet anxiety surrounding vaccines persists, as described in the smallpox chapter earlier in the book. In the 18th century people were frightened that vaccination might turn them into cattle, growing horns. Contemporary *Homo sapiens* is not free of equally mistaken conspiracy views, which can be seen as ways of dealing with uncertainty and anxiety about the unknown.

It is everyone's first question: Is it safe? The answer is a guarded yes. It is safe in pregnant women but wait for the second trimester; it is safe if you have antibodies but it should be avoided if you have allergies of any kind. The overwhelming majority of people want to have the vaccine and they should.

THE RUSSIAN INFLUENZA GLOBAL PANDEMIC OF 1889 TO 1892

As you look at the history of these coronavirus diseases, they seem to be increasing in viciousness. First trivial infections, then local epidemics with a significant mortality, escalating to a fulminating global pandemic. It may well be that overpopulation, urbanization, and change in farming techniques, as suggested by Shi Zhengli, are to blame. But this seeming "progression" from mild to severe may be an illusion.

The "Russian flu" of 1889–1892 was the first identified global pandemic to spread around the world in a year. It has been overshadowed in history by the Spanish flu that began thirty years later.

It started on the steppe in Uzbekistan, spread to St. Petersburg by train, and then continued around a planet newly connected by railways and steamships. It is estimated that it killed a million people—of the 1.5 billion on Earth. It spread with startling speed through the capitals of Europe. In England, Prince Eddy, Queen Victoria's grandson and second in line for the throne, caught the infection at the age of twenty-eight and died. The prime minister, Lord Salisbury, caught the infection and survived.

In the US, these events were eyed uneasily, and illusions of immunity disappeared when the pandemic devastated New York. It was the first city in the western hemisphere to be scourged by the Russian flu, and 13,000 died. It eventually was found on all the continents of Earth. Quinine was used in its treatment. The reason was simple; it was the only chemical compound known to cure an infectious disease. That disease was malaria and this disease was "flu," but surely it wouldn't hurt to try. Quinine lingered on as a treatment for flu and flu-like illnesses, particularly in Eastern Europe and the Far East, and it is an echo of this erstwhile therapy that led to the advocacy for hydroxychloroquine in SARS-Co-V2.

The Russian flu was worse in males and had a number of other features atypical for the usual flu. Diarrhea, neurological involvement, and particularly, a long convalescence with fatigue, pains in the joints, ringing in the ears, loss of taste, and depression were common.

Sound familiar?

The outbreak faded after six weeks, but the following winter it returned with equal virulence. Like the flu epidemics we have come to understand, it returned in the winter, but in the third year it was milder. Then it appeared to disappear but was actually lingering on as the common cold.

In 2005, Belgian virologist Leen Vijgen and her team showed that a virus that was causing an epidemic in cattle was a close genetic match to OC43, one of the four human coronaviruses discovered at the Common Cold Unit. By studying mutation rates, it was observed that these two similar viruses diverged in 1890 at the time of the Russian flu.

These findings suggest that the Russian flu pandemic was caused by a coronavirus that had spilled over from cattle to humans. It was virulent, as it had never been seen before, and the population was devoid of immunity. As time goes by, and through exposure, immunity develops and less virulent organisms have a survival advantage. The Russian flu evolved from being a global killer to the common cold. Perhaps there is more than one "flu" epidemic that was actually a coronavirus epidemic. Is it possible the other coronaviruses known to cause the common cold originated as a pandemic mistakenly called flu?

If this interesting speculation is applied to SARS-CoV-2, then it will also return in the winter months and decline in virulence over a few years to then become a minor infection.

CORONAVIRUSES: THE FUTURE

RNA viruses mutate all the time. We have seen with SARS-CoV-2 the advent of the UK variant and the South Africa variant. Don't forget that we only know this because for the first time we have been able to investigate a pandemic with powerful DNA/RNA technology.

This pandemic was predicted. We live in a cloud of RNA viruses. It is their increased mutation rate that allows these viruses to spill over into other species and then back into us. Coronavirus infections in animals other than humans are widespread. We have seen that massive numbers of coronaviruses are found in bats and a number of rodents throughout the world. They cause enteritis in cows and bronchitis in chickens. The disease goes from bats to pigs. Swine acute diarrhea syndrome (SADS) is a paroxysmal epidemic causing great economic inconvenience to pig farmers. Occasionally, humans are the intermediaries to animals. Shortly after the pandemic reached New York, five tigers and lions at the Bronx Zoo became sick with COVID-19. The intermediate hosts were zookeepers.

Yet mutation tends to lead to less virulent organisms. It is not in the interest of the virus to kill its host. Less virulence is a selective advantage. We have a misunderstanding here, let's work out a deal. This is how you would predict our relationship with coronaviruses would go. But the future has proved notoriously difficult to predict, has it not, and a new virulent virus could come at any time. There will be more pandemics and possibly more coronavirus pandemics, and it is to be hoped that what we have learned biologically and politically from this one will help us deal with the next.

CHAPTER 16

....

DISPATCHES FROM PANDEMICVILLE: COVID-19

We know that the significance of a pandemic at its onset is often played down with smug assurances from the authorities. Bubonic plague in San Francisco in 1900 and AIDS in New York in 1982 are two examples, and it was to happen again with SARS-CoV-2 in 2020.

I confess that I underestimated it—at the start, I thought it was just another flu.

MARCH 1, 2020—GATWICK AIRPORT, LONDON

An airport official asked me, "Have you been on mainland China in the preceding two weeks?"

"No."

I had heard of this distant outbreak but paid little attention. Flu comes from China every year. This one originated in a place called Wuhan.

On that packed transatlantic flight, there were an unusually high number of passengers wearing masks. About one in five. I thought that a bit excessive. It has long been established that airplanes carry viruses back and forth across the seven seas. Respiratory infections like colds and the flu predominate. More than a billion people travel by air each year, and a contagious person can travel anywhere on Earth within twelve hours. SARS-CoV-1 had traveled to Germany by air from 2002 to 2004. "That dwindled away," said my untroubled mind. We are culturally attuned to the flu. It's like malaria being hardly worth a second thought in West Africa. *One day, however, a serious pandemic is going to be spread everywhere by planes,* I thought without irony. I coughed inadvertently. The couple sitting to my right flinched.

After the plane landed at JFK, I read on my phone that by February 22, 2020, the disease had spread to Italy. As it was first detected in Chinese tourists there, the natural assumption was that it had been brought by plane. Did the flight I was on bring in a sample of the virus? By the time I got home to Woodstock, New York, all I wanted was sleep.

A Brief Timeline of COVID-19

- First cases reported in the world: Wuhan, China, December 31, 2019.
- First cases reported in Europe—France and Italy: January 15, 2020.
- First COVID-19 patient identified in the US: January 20, 2020, in Washington State. A man who had traveled from Wuhan.
- First COVID-19 patient in New York City: February 29, 2020. A man who had traveled from Italy.
- Within four months, the virus was to spread to every country in the world except for a few Pacific island states such as Tonga.

Other omens of what was to come had passed me by. Ten days after the outbreak had been reported to the WHO, on December 31, 2019, people were succumbing in Japan, South Korea, and Thailand. By January 7, 2020, Chinese scientists had isolated the virus and sequenced its RNA. It was a novel coronavirus, and this information was made available on the internet. That, I thought, was truly amazing.

MARCH 2, 2020—WOODSTOCK, NY

The phone rings. It is one of my three infectious disease colleagues welcoming me back. We chat. Then he goes on to tell me that we have a coronavirus patient.

"He's in the ICU on a ventilator. He's yours. We've divided the hospitals up between the group, and you've got Pandemicville."

I yawn. It's flu. I shower and get ready to go to work.

An elderly African American man is lying supine on an Intensive Care Unit (ICU) bed behind sliding glass doors. There is the usual transparent plastic tube sprouting out of his mouth connected to the ventilator. He is on an intravenous apparatus (IV), and there are monitor electrodes on his chest. His heart is beating fast. Nurse Mulligan is putting up a liter of saline. I think it's Nurse Mulligan. I can't quite tell, because she's encased in yellow with a yellow paper hat, yellow gloves, a blue N95 mask, and a second mask with a visor.

Outside the room, I ask, "What's the story?"

"His daughter had been in Italy," the resident tells me. "She flew back and drove to her dad's house here in upstate New York. She was coughing on the plane. The next day, she had a fever and felt terrible, so she called the Department of Health herself. Two men in HAZMAT suits met her in the parking lot of the hospital. They took nose swabs from her and her father and told them to quarantine themselves at home. It took forty-eight hours for the tests to come back. Both were positive for SARS-CoV-2. By the time she got the results, she was feeling better, but her father was feeling worse with a low-grade fever and he had lost his sense of smell."

We know what coronaviruses are (see Chapter 15). Each one is one-third the wavelength of light in size. Someone breathed on someone in China who breathed on someone in Thailand who took a plane to Italy who breathed on someone who breathed on this woman who breathed on her father who was now in the Pandemicville hospital ICU in the Hudson Valley with his very life under threat.

I gown up. While getting into my PPE, my mind has conjured an image of the well-known engraving of a plague doctor depicted during a bout of the bubonic plague in Europe in the 17th century. He is Dr.

Schnabel (Beak), and his long mask is filled with cloves and garlic. He's wearing a long black gown, a hat, and kid gloves, and is carrying a stick.

What does the patient think, already on the brink of delirium, when he sees Darth Vader—the new Dr. Beak—at the foot of his bed?

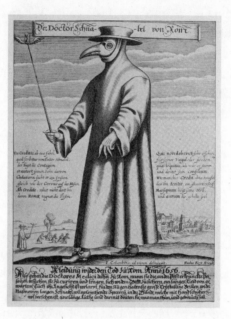

Copper engraving of Doctor Schnabel (Dr. Beak),
a plague doctor in 17th-century Rome, circa 1656.

The patient looks all of his eighty years. He is pale and sweaty, but alert. He's got a lowish blood pressure that's being maintained by intravenous medicines. I examine him. I am pessimistic. If I hadn't known about his coronavirus test, I would have said this was influenza pneumonia in an older man with age-weakened immunity.

I look up and wave at my two colleagues standing outside the room. I am in the room looking out, which has been the physician's place since before Hippocrates. Through plague, pandemic, infestation, scourge, and pestilence, we have been in the room looking out, and because of this, many physicians have lost their lives. I feel, for the first time, a little flicker of anxiety.

"Keep calm and carry on," an inner voice says.

Does a physician have a duty to treat? Death is an occupational hazard for doctors and nurses. The list is long, but here is one example: Six hundred American doctors lost their lives in the Spanish flu. In Pandemicville, the majority of docs have turned up for work as usual. My colleague Dr. Bert Ivanchik, a nephrologist, said, "Well, the nurses are here, why shouldn't I be?"

This is not the Spanish flu. At this point, the thinking goes, the overall mortality for this one will likely be much lower. And there's another reason this is not the Spanish flu: 102 years ago, we barely knew what viruses were. We didn't have effective treatment.

I take off my visor and put it on a flat surface. I take off my gloves, wash my hands, put on a new pair of gloves. I clean the visor with spirits, put the visor in a brown paper bag with my name on it. I take off the gloves, wash my hands, put on another new pair of gloves. I put my N95 face mask in a brown paper bag with my name on it and leave it with the other bag outside the room.

The team is comprised of a nurse, a respiratory therapist, an infectious disease doctor, and the intensivist. She is the physician in overall charge of this patient's management. We discuss treatment. We are in the process of getting into a trial of remdesivir, the drug that was used to treat Ebola. For now, we use an antiviral called Kaletra as well as hydroxychloroquine, an antimalarial. It's all empirical. There is no objective evidence that any of these treatments work.

It's the beginning of March.

What's next? There are many predictions, but reality will arrive one day at a time.

I look up. "Right," I say. "Who's free for lunch?"

MARCH 12, 2020—The ICU

Against all the odds, our first patient, let's call him Mr. First, is still alive. It's been a rocky course, but we are now weaning him off the ventilator. I give him a 50 percent chance of recovery. His daughter is beside herself with guilt for having brought the virus back with her from Italy. Relatives are now forbidden to visit and it's hard to reassure her on the phone. She shouldn't blame herself, but she does.

We have our temperatures taken when we come into the hospital in the morning. If it's normal we get a wristband. As soon as we cross the threshold, we put on disposable surgical masks and wear them all the time. When you reach the ICU, everyone is in scrubs. Personalized N95 masks are no longer kept in signed brown paper bags. They are thrown away safely and incinerated after one use. We are running out of N95 masks. All sixteen ICU beds have COVID-19 pneumonia patients, some on ventilators, and there's about twenty more in the hospital with the virus.

After pontificating to health care workers, supermarket salespeople, friends bumped into in the parking lot, and above all the CEO of the hospital, and asserting that flu killed forty thousand Americans last year, 10 percent of whom were young and healthy, and nobody insisted on social isolation for that or PPE, or taking our temperatures as we came into work, or any of the measures we have instituted, I have finally seen the light.

This is not the flu.

I called Luke Kelso, a friend working at Elmhurst Hospital in Queens, New York. As we spoke, I could hear sirens in the background. "We are at 110 percent capacity," he tells me. "Twelve people died yesterday of COVID-19. We have this guy here who was in Italy. He's saying, this is what it was like in Lombardy. We only have two intensivists and they can't cope. There are people on ventilators in the corridors. It's hitting the young, you know, forty-five to sixty age group. I'm supposed to be doing *obstetrics*, which has its own problems, as you can imagine—fever in labor . . . but mainly I help out in the ER."

I hear similar stories from Montefiore Hospital in the Bronx. The poor, the crowded together.

At the start of rounds that day, I say, "If I gave anyone the impression at any time that I thought that this was no different from flu, I was wrong. This isn't flu. This is NOT flu. The rate of death is far higher. In addition, there are clinical features of the disease that differ significantly from flu and that's what we are going to be talking about in a moment. And all through New York City there is carnage that you don't see with flu. Flu *non est. Mea culpa.*"

Why does this virus wreak such malevolence?

Technically, it doesn't actually wreak anything. It is a collection of molecules that know how to get into our cells, know how to replicate very efficiently once there, and know how to spread to infect other *Homo sapiens*. But that characterization is also completely wrong. They don't *know* anything. It's an astonishing accumulation of molecules that, in accordance with the principles of chemistry, act and interact in a random and valueless way leading to our infection and death. Do you see how difficult it is to talk about these little stinkers without projecting human qualities onto them? I just did it again. They don't even qualify as being *alive*.

We have come to understand earthquakes and tsunamis. We *get* asteroids crashing into the earth. We can probably figure out why blocks of masonry fall out of the sky on Fifth Avenue. But this? Something smaller than a wavelength of light? Such devastation?

We lost our fifth patient today. He had emigrated from Ireland at age sixteen. He ran a restaurant with his three sons. He was forty-eight. He had not knowingly been in contact with an infected person and he hadn't traveled to New York City, far less out of the country, for six years. He had a community-acquired infection. In other words, it infected him out of nowhere. He had a high fever from the start. A painful case.

There are about fourteen staff members running the unit. Stan the Nurse and I are the only males that day. Betty the Cleaner, covered in PPE, is swabbing out a recently emptied room. The nurses are going about their professional duties with effortless heroism and good humor. They have all turned up for work. No fuss. It's a normal day.

"When I get home at night, I undress in the garage," Nurse Mulligan says. "My boyfriend leaves a dressing gown and some slippers for me. When I come into the house, everyone else goes into the front room. We communicate by phone. I walk along the corridor and throw my clothes in the washing machine, remembering to turn it on. I walk upstairs and I take a shower. I love the shower! Then I dress. I bring the dressing gown back downstairs and throw it in the washing machine. And then . . . only then . . . the gin and tonic."

"Cytokine storm," says Janet, the intensivist, talking to her residents. "ARDS. We gave him hydroxychloroquine, azithromycin, zinc, vitamin D, vitamin C, anticoagulant. We gave him broad-spectrum antibiotics."

She leans against the console. She pauses, then returns to quizzing her two residents on how to treat ventilated patients.

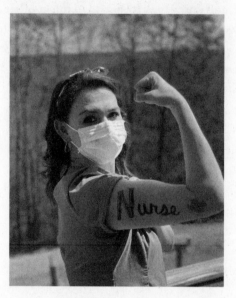

Nurse Rosy the Riveter.
Sara Oquendo, RN, photographic self-portrait.

FRIDAY, APRIL 3, 2020— PANDEMICVILLE HOSPITAL

The ICU is in a state of pandemonium. It is full and there are four more beds in opened storage rooms. We have nine COVID-19 patients on ventilators, seven on high flow oxygen. More nurses have been enlisted. The mood of the nurses is enthusiastic. Laughter predominates. One is shouting, two are speaking loudly.

I do my walk-around. Each room has a narrative. Its own opera.

In bed 6, the patient is twenty-two years old, obese, and doing badly. Like the Irishman, he had high fevers from the start. One hundred percent oxygen is not getting through his lungs to his bloodstream. Tests show his kidneys are failing. He has the numbers of death. Nurse Kim has just come out of the room divesting herself of PPE.

"He's dying," says Kim. "Dr. Janet says we are going to prone him, but he's a big guy; going to need three of us, I figure."

Dr. Janet, the intensivist, walks up. She is five feet tall and energetic.

She explains the physiology of proning. "See, if you place him facedown, the position of the heart and the diaphragm free up extra lung space through gravity. It can improve oxygenation. It is especially helpful in the fat."

"Don't you mean those with an increased basal metabolic index?"

"Are you getting politically correct with me? Have you put him on an antibiotic? He's got high fever and a high white count."

"I'm not convinced he has bacterial infection but wouldn't hesitate to give him broad-spectrum antibiotic. The white cell count is from the steroids."

"What are you gonna do? It makes sense, doesn't it, to soothe the cytokine storm?"

"True, but the steroids bring their own problems. It was in that article from Oxford, in the *New England Journal of Medicine*."

"Look, this guy is nearly gone, we have to try something. Now come in and help me prone this guy."

In any infection, there is an inflammatory response that is triggered by the immune system. You cut your finger, it gets infected, it gets red, painful, hot, and you can't use it properly. In serious body-wide infections such as septicemia, severe pancreatitis, and some infections such as flu and COVID-19, there is massive inflammation in the body. Too much inflammation. The inflammatory response starts hurting the body, not defending it. The chemical messengers in the blood that cause this are called cytokines. Thus, the cytokine storm. It starts to damage the lungs and leads to ARDS.

Mr. First, the eighty-year-old man who has been in the ICU for three weeks and whose daughter brought the virus from Italy, is still alive. He's no longer on the ventilator—an apparent victory—but he still requires high flow oxygen. He's tired and may not have the strength to breathe by himself much longer. Then what do we do? Put the tube back in? We must talk to his family.

I observe the scene. It's six thirty at night and it's busy like Grand Central Station. What am I saying? Grand Central Station is deserted. The on-the-floor activity is ordered. Some are gowning up; some are taking their gowns off. Some are working at computer terminals chatting energetically. It is really time to acclaim the nurses. There is M—I have never gotten on very well with her. Don't know why. Now, there she is, gowned up in the room answering written questions for a patient on high flow oxygen. I feel admiration for her and wonder in what way I have misunderstood her. Over these past few weeks, I have been privy to the Heroic—yes, with a capital *H*—the Heroic nurses. Across the hospital I have seen stoutheartedness, spirit, and class from these women. The nurses are mostly women, but we don't forget Stan and Eric.

Nurses are the superior branch of the health care team. It's all very well to turn out in the streets to applaud them as they are doing down in Brooklyn and Queens, but we should increase their pay. Without them, there would be no patient care at all. It is particularly so in the ICU.

Nurse Mulligan is caring for a fifty-four-year-old man who fled New York City. He brought his infection with him from Manhattan. She is in and out of his reverse, negative-pressure isolation room. Each time, she gowns up, pulls on her gloves, and puts on her HAZMAT visor. I watch her standing at his bedside, giving treatment through the IV. She cleans his face with a washcloth. She ups his oxygen a little. She checks his urine output. She keeps him clean in the bed. She writes some numbers on the whiteboard.

She removes her PPE in the anteroom and walks out into the main ward. "Hi, Doc!" she says. "Your N95 is upside down. You look like a hippo. Yeah, bed 12, he's shaping up. Oxygenating well, maintaining his BP. Did you hear what his wife calls the COVID-19? The boomer doomer. That's what they're calling it down in the city. He's looking really good."

The "boomer doomer"? Shall I laugh or cry? *When in doubt, laugh.*

The day ends. Not for the ICU—for me. On the way home, I stop to grab some takeout at a bistro-to-go.

"Hello, Doctor," says the man behind the counter.

Doctor? The other five people in the bistro shuffle away.

I pull into my driveway. One of my neighbors—wearing a mask—peers at me through a half-opened door. I blow her a kiss. She quickly closes the door. Settling into the socially distanced universe, I watch the news. Almost every country is dealing with the pandemic. So we really are a global village. We can be sure, therefore, that the governments of the world will put aside petty bickering and cheap political advantage and work together for the good of humanity!

Right.

There are no politics in the ICU.

THURSDAY, APRIL 17, 2020—
PANDEMICVILLE

I wake in Woodstock and drive to Pandemicville. Traffic is scarce. The hospital parking lot is half empty, but the Intensive Care Unit is packed double, maybe triple. I have never seen anything like this in my life, and this is not my first rodeo.

So, what exactly is going on? To recap: A collection of molecules one-third as large as the wavelength of light has been transmitted from a human in Wuhan, who coughed on another who passed it on to another, who traveled to Europe and coughed on another, then not just on to a man who traveled to upstate New York but infecting millions all over the world.

I know that this infinitesimally tiny virus has spikes on the outside, which slot perfectly into a well-known receptor found on the cell wall of the mucus membrane of the patient's inner nose, throat, and airway. It is called the angiotensin converting enzyme 2 receptor (ACE2) and it is associated with the regulation of blood pressure. We do not know how the virus evolved the ability to do that.

The RNA of the virus flows into the cytoplasm of the cell where it uses the cell's cellular factory to replicate the constituent parts of another virus, many more viruses each with a protein shell and RNA core, making new viruses that reassemble in the cell and burst out, a thousand, ten thousand going out for each one that entered, covered with spikes that will stick to the next ACE2 receptor they rub against.

It is, of course, more complicated than that. In molecular biological jargon, " . . . it entails ribosome frameshifting during genomic translation, the synthesis of genomic and multiple sub-genomic RNA species, and the assembly of progeny virions by a pathway unique among enveloped single-strand RNA viruses."

Diagnostic COVID-19 testing has been available from the start. Now antibody testing is available, which can determine if a person has had the disease in the past. My test is negative—to my disappointment. If you are positive and feeling well, you may have some immunity. If you are negative, you definitely have none. The picture is clouded, as asymptomatic positives may carry the virus and infect others. Research in this area is ongoing, but caution suggests positives should be quarantined even if feeling well.

To get to the ER, patients have to pass through a tent where physician assistants and nurses in full PPE assess them, then they progress to a second room where they may or may not be tested. Then they go to a specified area of the ER.

The only pandemic that comes close to this one, in terms of spread, is the Spanish flu of 1918. Both traveled by trains and boats, but only COVID-19 had the plane. When we consider future pandemics, we must think of this: How will we stop infected people, asymptomatic carriers, from getting on planes?

FROM THE GENERAL TO THE HUMAN

Mr. First, our eighty-year-old patient, is tiring. It has been four weeks. We feel that putting him back on the ventilator would only increase his suffering. When it comes to end-of-life matters, New York State law says that the wishes of the individual are paramount. It's up to *them* whether or not they wish to be resuscitated if their heart stops beating or whether or not they want to be intubated. But what do you do when the patient isn't capable of answering the question? If they've appointed a health care proxy, that person will make decisions on their behalf. It's not what the doctors want, nor what the family wants. The proxy is supposed to stay focused on *what the individual would have wanted*. It can be exceedingly difficult for a health care proxy to keep *his or her own* feelings out of the question. This is true of Mr. First's daughter.

Visitation by family members has been banned. With one exception: If the patient is dying, two visitors may come and make their farewells for half an hour. Mr. First's oldest son and his wife are at the bedside now in full PPE. Afterwards, we talk. They do not want him reintubated. They do not want him resuscitated if his heart should stop beating. But they don't want him to go on to palliative care with a morphine drip. They want us to treat him, give him high flow oxygen and other treatments, and let time make the decision for them. Abiding by the spirit and the letter of the law, this is what we will do. Inwardly, I think his chances of survival are nil.

Some patients come to the ICU and rapidly progress to death. They tend to be middle aged with an age range of forty-five to sixty-five. Similar patients look as if they are going to die but unexpectedly turn around. Risk factors, for any age group, are diabetes, hypertension, obesity, and gross immunocompromise such as patients on chemotherapy. It has been observed that people with blood group O do better than those with other blood groups and that blood group A does worst of all.

We are learning as we go. At the beginning of March, the dogma was to intubate early. Today, we avoid intubation for as long as possible. Medicines of uncertain value are prescribed less often. Hydroxychloroquine does not help, and if given with azithromycin, can hurt the heart, leading to abnormal rhythms. The question of using steroids or not is the subject of much debate. We treat on a case-by-case basis, but in the medical centers they only give drugs as part of a double-blind study. Half the patients get placebo.

The second patient we diagnosed—a seventy-year-old woman—had been in the ICU for four weeks. It seemed as if she were going to survive, but then suddenly she died. Why? Did she have a blood clot? A heart attack? An untreated infection? We wouldn't know without an autopsy. Her family did not consent.

I learn that Bert Ivanchik, my nephrologist friend, has tested positive and is currently at home. He is the first doctor in our hospital to come down with COVID-19. I call to check in.

"So, I'm feeling a bit tired," he says, "a bit achy. I drive home. My wife pours me a glass of wine. I go to smell the bouquet. What do I smell? *Nothing*. Get thee behind me, Anosmia. That's it. I say I've got the COVID. My temperature is 101 degrees Fahrenheit."

APRIL 21, 2020—WOODSTOCK AND PANDEMICVILLE

One time I thought I had been infected with SARS-CoV-2. It was a Wednesday afternoon, and I was cream crackered. That's London slang for very tired.

At three o'clock in the afternoon, I could barely drive home to my hut in the woods. I went to bed and instantly fell into a deep sleep. *Someone was talking to me faintly. I couldn't hear. Somebody whose voice I knew was telling me my fever was up, and just as a precaution I was being taken to the Intensive Care Unit for observation. "Just as a precaution," said the familiar voice from behind a mask and a visor.*

I saw a word written on the side of a trolley.

ISOLATION.

It said everything.

"We are going to give you a hundred liters of high flow oxygen and will only intubate you if absolutely necessary," said the voice bursting into song. Nessun dorma.

"Here comes Nurse Mulligan. She is going to pass a catheter," she says. Her eyes were smiling but she had an armful of writhing, hissing snakes.

When a child is born in Pandemicville hospital, Brahms's "Lullaby" is played on the PA. When a COVID-19 patient is discharged, they play "Don't Stop Believin'" by Journey, with lead vocalist Steve Perry.

Everyone stops and applauds when they hear that song. It wasn't playing often two weeks ago. More suggestions for a new theme song are made over a lunch of free Italian food that a local restaurant has donated to the staff of the ICU. "I Will Survive" by Gloria Gaynor. The anthem of the infectious disease confraternity is "Fever" by Peggy Lee. Other suggestions become increasingly tactless.

Mr. First is still alive. He is on less oxygen. So much so that they are thinking of moving him out of ICU down to the third floor, which is all under isolation. It's the SARS-CoV-2 ward. All PPE, all the time. It's nicknamed COVID Alley.

We have learned a number of lessons on COVID Alley about how the disease is different from flu in the following ways.

- There is variable onset. It is sometimes abrupt but more usually is subacute with people feeling unwell for a week or so before coming to the hospital.
- Mild diarrhea is not unusual; sometimes it is severe.
- Loss of the sense of smell and taste is not uncommon.
- Nearly everyone who is ill has fever with cough and breathlessness.
- The chest X-ray (CXR) shows patchy bilateral pneumonia. Often a computerized tomography (CT) scan of the chest is helpful in showing the characteristic ground-glass opacities. Radiologists will tell you this is more specific for identifying COVID-19 than a blood test.
- Secondary bacterial infection happens but is much less common than in flu.
- Patients live with lower oxygenation levels than has ever been seen before. They are called Happy Hypoxics and defeat my rudimentary knowledge of respiratory physiology.
- The infection causes a clotting disorder. One patient, a forty-year-old woman, presented with a classical blood clot in the lung from a venous clot in the legs. She tested positive for COVID-19. This tendency may account for some of the examples we see of sudden death. All patients are treated with blood thinners.
- Markers of inflammation are sky high. So, is it the immune response that kills? Yes, but that is the nature of all infectious diseases. They are interactions between microbe and immunity. As powerfully evolved as our immune system is, it is imperfect. Otherwise, we wouldn't get infections.
- Children under the age of ten are the least affected, but they are not unaffected. This is unusual. In most infectious diseases, children are particularly vulnerable. Their immunity is not fully formed and they suffer with the elderly, whose immunity is waning. This tells us we still have a lot to learn about the immunology of this interaction between a collection of molecules from out of thin air that know how to interact with our molecules in such an intimate and knowing way.

MAY 23, 2020—PANDEMICVILLE

I walk into the hospital. Someone pushes a gun into the middle of my forehead. It registers 98.2 degrees Fahrenheit. My previous wristband is cut off. A new one, color-coded for today, is put in its place. As this is happening, the overhead speaker starts to play "Don't Stop Believin'." I watch and applaud with the others as Mr. First is wheeled out of the hospital in a chair being pushed by his daughter. I wave. He waves back. Stay safe, Mr. First.

It's over. The COVID-19 pandemic is over. At least in the Hudson Valley of New York State. At least for now. We fear recurrence in the fall and winter. The ICU is half empty, but each bed holds a memory. Nurse Mulligan has handed in her notice. Her beau is a Texan and she is off to make a new life in Dallas.

MAY TO DECEMBER, 2020—USA

At first the hospital is half empty. Patients with the *'Vid*, as it's called in local slang, continue to arrive, but the number is down to a trickle. There is a fifty-year-old in the ICU who is very sick. We are doing our best to keep him off the ventilator. People with other standard internal medicine problems such as pneumonia or chest pain are scared to come to the hospital—to their detriment. Another example of the collateral ways the pandemic negatively affects our lives.

Bert Ivanchik had fever for three weeks, after which he returned to work. But he has not recovered. He is easily tired, still has no sense of smell, and has developed tinnitus, or ringing in the ears. I assure him this will pass. It's prolonged convalescence. People have started calling it Long COVID. It affects about one in twenty survivors and is worse in those who had severe disease. It is a mysterious entity. It is a syndrome known to complicate almost any infection, though rarely, and it may also occur after major surgery. Mononucleosis is notorious for causing it, and it looks like COVID-19 is going to be the same. Doctors have known about this since the Middle Ages, but what is happening in the body is not understood.

We watch the spread of the disease across the country and across the world. Mulligan reports from Dallas. She is up to her neck in it. I think she should receive the Congressional Medal of Honor. The US has the most cases and the highest death toll of any country in the world. More than 23.8 million infected, 400,000 dead. Are we absolutely certain we are not being punished by a wrathful God for some unspecified sin?

DECEMBER 2, 2020—PANDEMICVILLE

The number of admitted patients is on the rise. We have five patients in the ICU.

On November 26, Thanksgiving, 2,300 Americans died from COVID-19. It marks the first time that over two thousand people have died in a single day. The graph is going up. Los Angeles is going into lockdown. As winter comes, we fear we may return to the deep pandemic.

At the time of writing, 2 million have died in the world and 94 million have been infected.

CHAPTER 17

PLAGUES MAKE US
WHO WE ARE

W hat is life? Life is protein synthesizing replicating entities. We, the species *Homo sapiens*, replicate by sexual reproduction. Why?

Why do we replicate by sex? Is that even a question? And what, pray, has sex got to do with plagues?

Well, if it weren't for plagues, we wouldn't exist.

That is an impossible remark.

It's true.

THE BIOLOGICAL
INEFFICIENCIES OF SEX

At the beginning of your life, a sperm containing twenty-three chromosomes met an ovum also with twenty-three chromosomes. That's *you*, known at that point as a *zygote* with forty-six chromosomes, carrying your genes, to grow in the uterus of your mother.

Now, I don't intend any of what follows as a criticism of how we were all formed. We are talking in theoretical terms of what is biologically efficient. In whichever way I try to paint sexual reproduction as a negative, it must actually be a positive. That is the great conclusion of this argument.

What is the excellent benefit of sexual reproduction over this long list of apparent inefficiencies?

It would cost much less, biologically speaking, to replicate by binary fission, where the offspring has the same genes as the parent-entity. The individual just splits in two. Virgin birth or other ways in which uncomplicated life-forms can replicate without sex carries another version of this "benefit."

Let's look at the inefficiencies of sexual reproduction. First, the two-fold cost of sexual reproduction.

1. **Half of all offspring are male and cannot reproduce.**

   In poultry farming, chicken sexers are paid good salaries to distinguish between males and females at birth. Females lay eggs. A number of roosters are necessary to fertilize them and 1 or 2 percent would be plenty, but *50 percent*? For years, millions of male chicks were killed at birth. *Culled.* It is not even cost effective to grow them for meat. In recent years, this practice has been criticized, but the principle remains.

   Dairy farmers are in a similar financial bind. Bullocks are a drain on resources. At least you can grow them for food. "But please," implores the buttery man, "give me a heifer. They produce milk. They produce more cows."

   Now, when it comes to humans . . .

2. **Sexual reproduction leads to fewer offspring.**

   Sexually replicating females produce offspring at a lower rate than individuals that replicate by binary fission. Amebae double—then there are four, then eight, then sixteen. Humans have one child at a time. (With the exception of twins and triplets, of course.) Then another one. By the time a human mother has had five children, the asexual creature has sixteen. Two who multiply by parthenogenesis will have twice as many children as a man and a woman.

There are more inefficiencies in human sexual reproduction.

- The species must evolve the anatomical apparatus for reproduction.
- Menstruation is required, leaving females infertile two to seven days a month. Menopause is another biological inefficiency.
- Ova and sperm have only twenty-three chromosomes and are known as germ cells. All other cells have forty-six. A means was evolved to reduce the number of genes in these cells by half, a process known as *meiosis*. It takes place in the reproductive organs, but why did this complexity have to evolve? The energy involved in evolving meiosis is enormous. If you multiplied by binary fission, it wouldn't be needed.
- Dating. The complexities of finding a date are not new. This is not trivial. There are pragmatic problems in the mammalian world that binary fission does not have to deal with, including male competition.
- Loss of favorable genes in the mixing process.
- Sexually transmitted diseases.
- Waste of biological resources evolved for conception.
- Diseases of the newly evolved sex organs. The three most common cancers of women are breast, ovary, and uterus. Infection of the sex organs can only occur in species that practice sexual reproduction.

Sex started about two billion years ago. It is still popular. And, to be fair, it is not just us—99 percent of multicellular creatures reproduce sexually. But why? From the costs outlined above, you would think it a losing enterprise. It must have a huge benefit to overcome these drawbacks.

What is it?

BREEDING LIKE . . . RABBITS

In 1787, the First Fleet departed England to settle in Australia and took six male and six female rabbits with them. The gestation period of a rabbit is thirty-one days. By 1950, there were several hundred million rabbits destroying crops all over the continent. Myxomatosis virus, harmless to *Homo sapiens*, was given to the bunnies and killed 99.8 percent of them by an acute infectious disease not dissimilar to measles. A few rabbits were infected by mosquitos and then it became transmissible from rabbit to rabbit.

Which means that, of a hundred million, two thousand survived.

Rabbits sexually reproduce, which leads to the mixing of male and female genes. This coming together of specific males with specific females, known as *dioecious* sex, means there will be some rabbits with genes, among an almost infinite variety, that have innate resistance to myxomatosis. This enables them to survive and to pass on their innate resistance to their offspring.

If all rabbits had identical genes, which would be the case had they multiplied by binary fission or parthenogenesis, *all* would have died. In sexual reproduction, the offspring is not identical to the mother; when the next wave of myxomatosis comes along, more rabbits will have genetic resistance to the infection and fewer will die.

Individuals that asexually reproduce have a hundred identical lottery tickets. Individuals who sexually reproduce have fifty different ones with a much better chance of giving birth to offspring that will resist infection and survive.

By the year 2000 in Australia, there were as many rabbits as before, and they were all immune to the myxomatosis virus. There is something else to consider regarding the survival of the rabbits. It is not in the interest of the virus to kill its host, as it would therefore kill itself. When random mutation produces a less virulent virus, it is selected because it survives longer. The virus shares a common interest with us. Pathogens tend to become less virulent over time. Virulence is a sign of novelty. A good example of this is the coronavirus SARS-CoV-2.

This co-evolution between pathogen and host will have happened over and over again in our animal ancestors and in ourselves. Past plagues are written in our genomes. Plagues never kill everyone. Amid the huge mortality of the Inuit from influenza, a few survived. The eventual mortality of AIDS, before antiretroviral drugs, was not 100 percent but 96 percent. All plagues have survivors. It is one reason why, despite the twelve plagues described in this book, and their appalling mortalities, the population of humans on Earth has gone up from 3.7 billion in 1970 to 7.6 billion in 2020, doubling in a mere fifty years.

Animals are usually killed by other creatures: parasites, predators, and competitors. The First World War killed twenty-five million people in four years; the Spanish flu killed eighty million or more in one.

In our world, two individuals, by having sex, can produce offspring who are more likely to survive than an individual that produces clones of itself. In a world without infectious diseases, asexual reproduction would prevail. It is so much more efficient.

Efficient though it is, asexual reproduction has a huge drawback. It allows harmful mutations to persist, leading in most cases to extinction after about two hundred generations. So, if it were not for plagues, we would not exist. Plagues were and are the evolutionary pressure that led to sexual reproduction. *If it were not for plagues, we would not exist.*

Sexual reproduction allows genes to mix, leading to diversification. It facilitates a staggering level of variability among genes that code for the proteins of immunity. These proteins play a crucial role in the adaptive branch of the immune system. There is such a wide variety among the population that someone will survive whatever comes our way. Some will survive SARS-CoV-2. Others will survive HIV. Still others will survive the Spanish influenza. These genes form what is known as the major histocompatibility complex, or MHC, and can vary enormously among individuals. This variability is called *polymorphism*, and you are more likely to have the same fingerprints as another person than the same MHC genes.

Infectious diseases are caused by relentless, insatiable microbes that would have extirpated us had we not evolved the immune response, including an enormous diversity of genetic resistance genes so that whenever a plague hits, there will be some with genetic resistance who will survive to replicate.

If genetic diversity through sexual reproduction leads to resistance to, and survival from, disease, how have the bdelloid rotifers that have been replicating by binary fission, that is asexually, survived for eighty million years? Well, under times of stress and pathogenic infection, they are able to desiccate themselves and are blown away in the wind. They then reassemble elsewhere. This would not work for you and me. We can't desiccate.

So, we depend on sexual reproduction, thanks to infectious diseases, for our survival.

But what if a plague killed us all? Happily, as we've seen, it would have to overcome the polymorphism of the MHC, of the adaptive immune response, and so far, that hasn't happened.

Romeo and Juliet. Dr. Zhivago. *All the great love stories are, in the last analysis, just because of the inexorable presence of plagues?*

Yes.

So, what you are saying is, relationships, sleepless nights, mad excitement, love songs, wolf whistles, movies, pornography, dancing, the Trojan War, Jane Austen, Marilyn Monroe . . . are all there so we can mix our genes? So that some of us can survive the next plague?

Exactly.

INFECTIONS SHAPE OUR GENES

In the past, plagues may have been thought of as random misfortunes that popped up from time to time like hurricanes, or volcanoes erupting, but we should not be thinking that way now. Plagues are not caused by microbes "doing" something to us, they are an interaction between them and us. We share our body space with more bacteria than we have cells, and viruses make up nearly 50 percent of our genes. We could not have evolved without the mitochondrion, a symbiotic bacterium living in every one of our cells. This long association with relatively harmless microbes is one part of our biology. Our interactions with microbes that cause disease have led to another huge area of our biology—immunity. Microbes have determined the biochemistry of our bodies and the necessity for sexual reproduction to mix genes and ensure our survival. Our intimate, biological association with microbes doesn't stop there. They also shape our genes.

Sickle cell disease (SCD) is a curse. It is an inherited disease that causes the formation of abnormal hemoglobin, the molecule that carries oxygen around the body in red blood cells. Under the microscope, this abnormal hemoglobin looks like little sickles—normal cells are disc-shaped—and turns the red cells into sludge. SCD leads to anemia, painful bone and abdominal crises, predisposition to infection, blood clots leading to stroke and worse, all accompanied by diminished fertility, and, with the best care, a life span of forty years.

The gene that is the DNA code for the protein hemoglobin resides on human chromosome 11 in all of us as well as in all of our cells. The gene codes for 574 amino acids and the one at position 6 in those without sickle cell disease (nearly all of us) is glutamic acid, the DNA code for which is G-A-G. In sickle cell disease, glutamic acid is replaced by valine, the code for which is G-T-G. That's it, swap a T for A and you have the disease. One base pair difference in three billion base pairs leads to sickle cell disease. According to Darwin, mutations occur randomly and most of them are "bad" for the organism. G-A-G to G-T-G is such a mutation. So, how is it that sickle cell disease is one of the most commonly inherited diseases in the world and the number of people suffering from it is increasing?

Sickle cell disease is a recessive disorder, meaning that two abnormal genes, one from each parent, are necessary to cause the disease. If you have a sickle cell gene from one parent and a normal one from the other, you are a carrier. The biological word for carrier is *heterozygote*. Those with the disease are *homozygotes*.

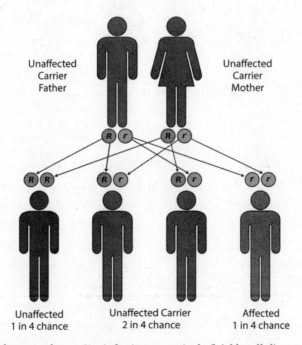

Autosomal recessive inheritance typical of sickle cell disease.
Cburnett via Wikimedia.

Consider the diagram above. If two carriers mate, one in four of their offspring will have SCD. Two in four will be carriers. One in four will neither have the disease nor be a carrier. Carriers are *immune to malaria*. That is why the disease persists in the malaria zone. Stated in biological terms: In the presence of malaria, SCD continues to exist at a high rate as the heterozygote carrier state gives a selective advantage to the population.

The WHO map below shows that a preponderance of the global incidence of malaria is in sub-Saharan Africa. There are over a hundred countries with people who have the disease. It is estimated that there are 0.5 million people born yearly with SCD and 5.5 million carriers in malaria endemic zones.

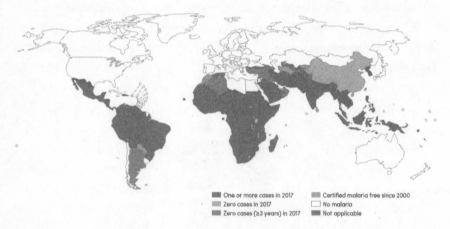

One or more cases in 2017   Certified malaria free since 2000
Zero cases in 2017   No malaria
Zero cases (≥3 years) in 2017   Not applicable

WHO map showing the preponderance of malaria.

Imagine you are a carrier living in a malaria zone and you wish to have children with another carrier. Mother Nature has a deal for you. Half of your children will be immune to malaria because they have sickle cell trait. One in four will not have the disease but would be vulnerable to malaria with a 10 percent mortality. But, because of the way genetic odds work, one in four of your children will die a prolonged and painful death over ten to thirty years because of SCD. Mother Nature pursues a course, not very maternally, where the benefit to the species outweighs the suffering of an individual.

But now let's look at this situation from another angle. Twenty percent of the eleven million slaves imported from West Africa to America between 1540 and 1888 carried the gene for SCD. Which explains why, in 2018, SCD affects one hundred thousand Americans, with two million carriers. One in thirteen African Americans is born a carrier.

One in 365 African Americans has the disease.

One in 16,300 Hispanic Americans has the disease.

Malaria has disappeared in America, but sickle cell remains. In the US, there is presently no benefit to being a carrier with sickle cell trait. In the absence of malaria, the sickle cell gene has no selective advantage and should theoretically disappear. It will, but at a very slow rate. In the US, the incidence is falling by about 0.01 percent per year. If you are an American carrier, would you have children with another American carrier?

Without the protection from malaria it provides to carriers, sickle cell disease appears to be a cruel trick of fate. Imagine there was no knowledge of the disease of malaria in the United States—no textbook description, no literary account, nothing. On top of that, there is neither knowledge nor history of the slave trade. It has been lost. Or it was never recorded. The disease would be classified as a genetic disorder of unknown causes.

Sickle cell disease is not the only abnormality that exists because of malaria. These genetically inherited diseases occur in at least five hundred million people, yet when they are carriers, they survive malaria. This shows how diseases—in this case malaria alone—have shaped the human genome.

Other disorders that inherently have protection from malaria include:

- Alpha thallasemia
- Beta thallasemia
- Hemoglobin C trait
- Hemoglobin E trait
- Glucose-6-phosphate dehydrogenase deficiency
- Pyruvate kinase deficiency
- Elliptocytosis
- Ovalocytosis (which is common in Southeast Asia)
- Persistence of fetal hemoglobin

- Specific human leukocyte antigen (HLA) tissue types
- Duffy antigen negativity with five other similar genetic variations

There is another malaria connection in this group of disorders. Duffy antigen negativity protects against *Plasmodium vivax*, the second most common cause of malaria. *Vivax* causes a milder disease than that caused by *falciparum*. It also evolved in Africa and jumped into *Homo sapiens* on the continent, yet it is not found there. *Vivax* can only enter the red cell through the Duffy receptor, a protein found on red cells. A mutation occurred, where no Duffy receptor appeared on the red cell of one human. So beneficial was this occurrence that a few hundreds of thousands of years later, the overwhelming majority of Africans and their descendants have no Duffy receptor and are immune to *Plasmodium vivax* malaria, unlike those without the mutation. However, there is a cost because Duffy-negative Africans are more prone to getting AIDS. Although, if they do acquire AIDS, they live longer than those who are Duffy positive.

Note, sickle cell *disease* itself tells us nothing about the nature of malaria. Did other genetic disorders evolve as protection against unknown infectious diseases?

SEARCHING FOR HETEROZYGOTES: FROM THE ASHKENAZIM TO THE IRISH

The Ashkenazi Jews originally lived in central and northern continental Europe. Their culture has changed little since they came into being somewhere between the beginning of the 13th century and the end of the 15th. They are descended from as few as 350 individuals. It is unknown why so few, but they could be survivors of a catastrophe, man-made or climatic. Or they could represent a small group that broke off from a larger group for any number of reasons, including religion. Ashkenazim tend to live isolated from other populations and have large families with a high incidence of cousin marriages.

Before the Famine of 1848, most of the Irish beyond the Dublin Pale were peasant farmers living in poverty, over-dependent on the potato yet increasing in population at a great rate. One county, Clare, saw its population double to three hundred thousand in twenty years before the famine. That's about three times County Clare's population in 2020. Cousin marriages were frequent in this population.

These two diverse cultures both characteristically have large families and cousin marriages. They also have high numbers of and many types of autosomal recessive inherited genetic disorders. First cousins share 12.5 percent of their genetic material and are more likely to inherit the same mutation from a common ancestor. More remote cousins, although having fewer genes in common, still have more shared genetic material than unrelated people.

NIEMANN-PICK C1 DISEASE

With this disorder, fats are not broken down and they accumulate in the organs of the body, particularly the brain. Homozygotes have nervous system and skin involvement, and most die in childhood. The disease is found in all societies so far examined but is most common in the Ashkenazim.

Both heterozygotes and homozygotes are missing a receptor to the cell, which is the same one that filoviruses such as Ebola use to enter. If you have Neimann-Pick disease or if you are a carrier, you can never get Ebola!

As far as anyone knows, the Ashkenazim have never been submitted to severe evolutionary pressure from this lethal infection, as is the case with malaria and sickle cell disease. There may be other viruses that we know nothing of that enter the cell this way; or it may be the simple intervention of chance.

CYSTIC FIBROSIS (CF)

One in nineteen Irish people are heterozygotes for cystic fibrosis (CF), the highest rate known in the world. Among the Ashkenazim, the rate is one in twenty-four. CF is the most common lethal single-gene mutation in people of European descent. The fundamental defect is a mutation in the gene that allows for transport of fluid and ions from cell to cell, leading to sticky secretions that cause early and persistent lung infections. Later, those with CF may develop liver and pancreatic disease.

Early suggestions of what lethal infectious disease CF carriers might be protected against were cholera and typhoid, but these have been disproved by epidemiological studies and bench science experiments on mice. Epidemiological evidence strongly supports the hypothesis that cystic fibrosis carriers of the CF gene are protected against tuberculosis. In addition, the tuberculosis pandemic, accelerating in 17th-century Europe, occurred at the right time and place to select for CF. So lethal was tuberculosis that a resistance rate of only 13 percent would be of sufficient benefit to explain the frequency of the cystic fibrosis gene.

CCR5

CCR5 is a receptor for chemokines on the cell membrane of a number of cells, particularly the CD4 lymphocyte (a white blood cell). It is part of the incredibly complex human immune system. The CD4 lymphocyte is also the cell infected by HIV, and its destruction leads to the severe immunodeficiency of AIDS. For HIV to enter a cell, it must bind to two protein receptors on the cell's membrane, CD4 and CCR5. You can think of CD4 as the lock and CCR5 as the key. If CCR5 is missing, the virus cannot enter the cell. If it can't enter the cell, that person cannot get AIDS.

Now, as it happens, CCR5 is missing in some humans. This mutation happened about 1,200 years ago. It arose in Northern Europe at the time of the Vikings. Today, about 16 percent of Finns to 4 percent of Sardinians cannot acquire AIDS because of the absence of CCR5. Absence of CCR5 has not been described outside of Europe.

Therefore, these people are naturally immune to AIDS. As incredible as this is, the mutation couldn't have arisen in response to AIDS. There was no AIDS in any parts of Europe 1,200 years ago. In the absence of a selective pressure, a single mutation would typically take 127,500 years to reach 10 percent of a population. Here it took a thousand years. So, if HIV was not the selective pressure that led to this frequency, what was? The other virus that enters the cell through CCR5 is smallpox. All evidence suggests that the mutation arrived by chance and was then encouraged to survive by the advantage it gave against smallpox.

Vikings sailing down the Rhine bent on rape and plunder could merrily accomplish their pillaging because they were immune to smallpox. CCR5 is inherited in a dominant fashion, so three-quarters of a Viking's offspring would have the gene, and one day, fifty generations down the line, the descendants would be immune to HIV infection. And, incidentally, as a bonus, absence of CCR5 also protects against cerebral malaria, although not the other forms of the disease.

But in the never-ending tug-of-war between host and infectious agent, an absence of CCR5 makes you *more* susceptible to infection with West Nile virus. It should come as no surprise that the CCR5 receptor and its absence are currently the subject of a vast area of research across many fields.

––––––––––

There are 345 autosomal recessive genetic diseases recognized worldwide to date, and new ones are being discovered. The genetic screening of a thousand Saudi families in 2016 revealed five never-before described diseases and twenty-seven candidate autosomal recessive genes. There are already a much larger number of autosomal recessive disorders among the Saudis than Europeans. Protection from an infectious disease is not the only explanation for an increased number of autosomal recessive disorders in a community, but it must account for some.

An infection is not just a protist, bacteria, or virus visiting disease upon us; our genetic makeup is an unindicted co-conspirator in the illness. In the presence of healthy immunity, it is the two together that will determine the severity of the infection and the course it takes.

CHAPTER 18

. . . .

WHAT PLAGUES
MAY COME

A pandemic is a misunderstanding between microbe and host. As everyone is now fully aware, there will be more misunderstandings. When they will occur and how they will unfold is more difficult to determine. How can we prepare?

To be writing a book about plagues when a novel pandemic arrives to afflict the whole world is an uncommon experience. It sheds light on the plagues of history at a time when previous plagues can illuminate this one. Our knowledge of microbes in general, viruses in particular, as well as of epidemiology and social hygiene, is more complete now than ever. So, how did that knowledge improve our response to SARS-CoV-2, the virus that causes COVID-19? Not as much as we might have hoped.

Literate educated societies behaved in the 21st century as illiterate uneducated societies did in the 17th. Man, the impossible primate, must understand that compulsions to denial, tribalism, xenophobia, conspiracy theories, and scapegoating in a plague will only increase the number who die.

There are two particular areas where we need to improve our game. First, we must understand that pandemics are not caused by viruses or bacteria alone. They are structured, spread, and nurtured by ourselves, *Homo sapiens*, the victims. This has to guide our policies.

Second, in the history of plagues, politicians have nearly always got things wrong. When bubonic plague hit London in 1605, a halfpenny was paid by the elders of the City of London to anyone who killed a stray dog because it was widely "understood" that dogs spread the disease. They didn't. What dogs were best at was keeping the rat population down.

The trouble is, the cost of a plague is enormous. It is not just the cost of treatment as we veterans of COVID-19 are only too well aware; it is job loss, business failure, and loss of savings. Plagues are terrible for business. What sacrifices are we prepared to make to preserve it? Leaders are thrown into conflict over how to balance the economy versus health. Herd immunity! There's an idea. The more people that get infected, the more quickly we will attain herd immunity. Of course, this is going to cost the lives of x number of people. *Hmmm. Maybe it's okay if someone else's grandparents or other loved ones die? But wait a minute...* Such ideas are morally untenable, and we know it, but valuable time is lost in contemplating the issue.

If only we listened more to the experts. We must forget the Health of the Economy until we have an Economy of Health. Mastering these issues is of great importance, as the threat of a new global pandemic is at least as great as it ever was and may be greater.

Modern-day Cassandras, often scientific experts, who have predicted the coming of plagues, are ignored. There are underestimations, cover-ups, lies, blame-mongering, and scapegoating. The actions of invisible little creatures leading to our deaths belongs to the animal side of our nature, that thing we don't like to talk about. We pretend it isn't there.

Plagues spread at the speed of the available transport. The question of where they will originate is important, but less so, because they can start anywhere on Earth and be taken everywhere. Most plagues spill over from animals. Plagues in *Homo sapiens* are increasingly caused by viruses, as was the case with the three major plagues of the 20th century—Spanish flu, AIDS, and smallpox. SARS-CoV-2 is also viral. Three of these are spillover pandemics. Smallpox is the exception but that too could be a spillover; it's just that the putative animal from which it spilled has not been identified.

There are approximately three hundred pathogens that infect us, an infinitesimally tiny percentage of the number of species of bacteria, virus, protozoa, fungus, and worms on Earth. Viruses are everywhere, and we couldn't live without them. Bacteria are everywhere, and we couldn't live without them, either. Viruses are literally in our genes and have dominated our history and our bodily structure. As we saw in Chapter 17, sexual reproduction is a defensive adaptation to plagues. Our genome has been arranged to deal with virulent pathogens by developing structural, non-infectious diseases like sickle cell disease, cystic fibrosis, and other genetic disorders whose infectious origin may never be discovered. Our interaction with pathogens has always been the most powerful single factor driving human evolution.

One generalization that can be made about pandemics is that we tend to ignore the last one. When the new one comes along, only then do we acknowledge the last one and pore over it for insights. In 2020, interest in the Spanish flu has skyrocketed.

In *Gone with the Wind*, Scarlett O'Hara's first husband, Charles Hamilton, died in the Civil War. Did he distinguish himself in valor on the battlefield? No. In a failure of manliness, Hamilton died from the measles. Dying of Spanish flu in the First World War would have been equally humiliating. We're titillated and inspired by death, glory, courage, betrayal, politics, and action-filled stories. The death certificates of American soldiers who died from the flu often had *Killed in Action* put as the cause of death as an act of compassion to the family. Historians have often diminished the dominating consequences of plagues, except for a select minority who specialize in their study. This *was* true—until now.

LEARNING FROM EBOLA?

In December 2013, there was an outbreak of Ebola virus infection, primarily in West Africa. Eleven thousand people died over the course of three years in Guinea, Liberia, and adjacent countries. United States president Obama called it the Ebola *crisis*. This declaration was followed by panic. Ebola is a contagious viral infection with a high mortality rate, and what unfolded in West Africa was indisputably a tragedy. Of course, the death rate from Ebola doesn't come close to the number of people dying there yearly of malaria, tuberculosis, and measles, which are preventable diseases, but Ebola is a singular outbreak that deserves our scientific attention and it is natural and correct to be concerned about controlling its spread. That is not what happened.

What unfolded in America in response was a bizarre eruption of hysteria, conspiracy theory, and absurdity that stood in sharp and strange contrast to the silence that greeted Spanish flu for fifty years after World War I. It is worth observing that few politicians or pundits paid the slightest attention to the experts in the field; they ignored the virologists and epidemiologists whose life work was the study of the ways of dealing with viral epidemics like Ebola, areas of expertise in which the US led and still leads the world.

Catching Ebola required contact with bodily secretions of the infected. It is not transmitted by coughing. It is not transmitted through the air. The views of the experts were ignored concerning transmission, and, indeed, on everything else surrounding the disease. Panic prevailed. In an attempt to combat the "threat" of Ebola, a sad level of geographic obliviousness was revealed. People who were in the US from Zambia and South Africa, countries two thousand or more miles away from the epidemic in West Africa, were sent home. Schools denied scholarships to Nigerians. Although they were from a country with a population of 120 million and nine cases of Ebola, suddenly they were unwelcome out of an "abundance of caution." On the door of a blood test lab in Kingston, New York, was a sign: "If you have recently been to Africa, Do Not Enter." Conspiracy theories spread across the internet and were seriously touted on cable TV: President Obama apparently wanted Ebola to infect white Americans as payback for slavery; it was a terrorist threat and immigrants were deliberately bringing it across the borders.

Over the strenuous objections of many, seven infected American missionaries were flown to the United States from Liberia for treatment. The prevailing attitude was: "They should accept the consequences. They should not have gone to work in African cesspools." Never was sainthood held in such low esteem. Fortunately, such views were ignored and all seven were treated and survived.

Two Liberians brought the disease to Texas and died. Two nurses acquired Ebola from looking after these patients; both survived. So, of eleven people with the disease on American soil, two died. No new cases have been seen in the United States since the last patient was released from the hospital on November 11, 2014. Once it was clear that the danger was gone, the subject was dropped like a stone. Except, of course, by those same virologists and epidemiologists who appear to have found a cure in 2019 (see Chapter 14).

So, it seems we can underreact, overreact, but can never get it quite right.

In spite of plagues, our species is growing in number. Some 7.8 billion *Homo sapiens* live on the planet, as of 2020. In 1960, the total was 3.03 billion. This is great biological success for the species but is not so great when considering the costs and risks entailed in that growth: destruction of the environment and *Homo sapiens'* penchant for war.

When it comes to epidemic illnesses, however, the end of the world is not necessarily nigh. We have made some progress. On the positive side, medicine saves endangered lives. Science has given us the means to study microbes that cause plagues, provided some treatments, and, in the case of COVID-19, produced a vaccine within a year of the first cases being reported.

We must find the viruses before they find us.

We enter the rain forest where the pathogens live, we live in large cities where we incubate them, and we fly around the world disseminating them. But there are things that can be done. A seven-pronged program would go a long way to curtailing risk:

- Stop destroying the rain forests.
- Stop global warming.
- Support vaccine research and encourage its use around the world.
- Provide clean drinking water for all, as in the WASH initiative (Water, Sanitation, and Hygiene—a UNICEF program).
- Support scientific and pharmaceutical research.
- Continue strengthening our monitoring ability through the WHO and the Centers for Disease Control and Prevention.
- Educate.

All these approaches are important, but a little bit *more* is needed. In 1808, 1811, and 1817, in the village of Wimbledon outside of London, there were outbreaks of smallpox. Mr. Sanford, an apothecary, each year requested of the burghers of the village that the poor of the parish be given the "cow-pock" vaccination, as indicated by Edward Jenner, in spite of the cost. It was £70 in the first year, £18 15s at the second outbreak, and £45 in 1817. Agreement was unanimous. They coughed up the funding at once. Did they care that much about the poor? Did they have to overcome a feeling that it was not their responsibility to pay for other people's health care? Or did vaccinating the poor lower the smallpox risk to their own children and themselves? At the end of the day, it was enlightened self-interest that led to "protection for all."

And it may be in this sentiment that the mastery of plagues really begins.

EPILOGUE:
WHERE ARE
THEY NOW?

We described twelve plagues, but there are many more. Leprosy, measles, and poliomyelitis immediately come to mind. But considering our rogue's gallery of eleven and COVID-19, with the exception of smallpox, the lot are as globally active as ever. Even as we fear new plagues, we continue to suffer from the old ones. Indeed, the number afflicted are greater than ever before, attributable primarily to the increase in population.

1. **Bubonic plague**

   One to three thousand new cases are reported in the world every year for the last decade. These days, epidemic plague tends to occur in rural settings, with flare-ups, as have occurred in Central Africa, Eastern Eurasia, and China particularly. The disease also simmers at a low level in the Andes and the six southwestern states of the United States. The island of Madagascar is endemic for plague with yearly flare-ups in the summer months from November to April. In 2016, 2,400 people acquired the disease with a 25 percent mortality. Of these, 75 percent had the pneumonic form of plague. Those affected live mostly in the capital. There is no plague, from 1950 to the present, in Europe, Australia, or New Zealand.

2. Cholera

Although cholera was noted in Yemen in 1970–1990, it had disappeared in 1990–2004. Yet, in October 2016, the worst cholera outbreak in recorded history began in that country. More than two years of fighting between the Saudi-led coalition and the Houthi rebels had displaced large numbers of people, destroyed access to clean water and sanitation, and driven millions to the brink of famine. An estimated one and a half million people have died. This is a medieval-level catastrophe in the 21st century. Cholera became epidemic in Haiti following an earthquake in 2010, for the next seven years. In a lesson to be taken in the spread of epidemics, the origin was found to be peacekeeping forces from Nepal. It would not have spread without the collapse of infrastructure, overcrowding, and poverty. The lessons are: War continues to breed epidemics, and global travel spreads diseases more efficiently than ever before.

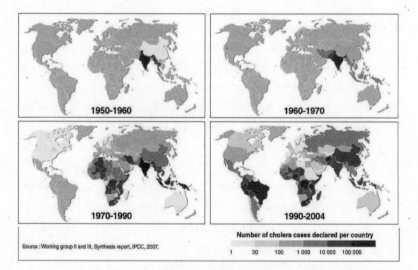

Distribution of cholera.
The darker the shade, the more cholera. Image by IPCC.

3. **Typhus**

In 2018, there was an outbreak in Los Angeles County, when fifty-seven cases of flea-born typhus were recorded. The primary vector is usually rats or mice. The number of actual infections may well be much higher because mild bouts are common and are often diagnosed as something else. Typhus persists worldwide, but major outbreaks are usually found in association with war. *Rickettsial* infections are flourishing around the world for the same reason as mosquito-borne infections—the insect vectors are increasing and uncontrolled.

4. **Tuberculosis**

One in three of the world's population, two and a half billion people, are infected with tuberculosis in its latent form. Of those, nine million become sick with the disease and one and a half million people die every year. About four million people died of tuberculosis in the United Kingdom in the second half of the 19th century, but tuberculosis continues to infect as many people in the world as ever. Countries in sub-Saharan Africa and the Far East have the highest burden. It is the most common cause of death in those afflicted with AIDS. European and North American countries have learned how to screen for, diagnose, and treat the infection. However, multi-drug resistant strains (MDR) and extra-drug resistant strains (XDR) already exist and are seen in most countries afflicted with the disease. Resistance is being countered with the development of new antibiotics, so the biological arms race will continue.

5. **Syphilis**

The WHO reported in June 2019 that one million new cases of curable sexually transmitted infections—gonorrhea, chlamydia, trichomoniasis, and syphilis—were transmitted daily among people aged fifteen to forty-nine. That's 376 million new cases annually. The number of annual cases of syphilis is seven million, and these numbers are the same as the last published data from 2012. It causes an estimated two hundred thousand annual stillbirths, with congenital syphilis in those who survive. The most effective treatment is in short supply as there is a global shortage of benzathine penicillin. The syphilis bacteria *Treponema pallidum* has developed resistance to macrolide antibiotics but not penicillin. There is rapidly increasing resistance of *Neisseria gonorrhea* to antibiotics.

6. **Malaria**
The World Health Organization has vowed to eliminate the disease, as has philanthropist Bill Gates. Each year the malaria parasite kills 830,000. Eradication of malaria has been a goal since the 1950s. Current evidence suggests that the partial success gained over the last twenty years is again waning.

7. **Smallpox**
Eradicated from the world in December 1979. The only other plague to be eradicated is rinderpest in cattle, a measles-like viral infection. Measles in humans has not been eradicated.

8. **Yellow fever**
Forty-seven countries in Africa and Central and South America are endemic for, or have regions that are endemic for, yellow fever. They and their neighbors will not allow entry without evidence of vaccination. Because there is a safe and effective vaccine for the disease, there is the Eliminate Yellow Fever Epidemics (EYE) strategy of the WHO to prevent, detect, and respond to yellow fever epidemics in at-risk countries. It is estimated that more than a billion people will have been vaccinated by 2019. The trouble is, there are often marked international shortages

of vaccine for uncertain reasons. As of 2020, there are current outbreaks in Angola and Brazil.

9. **Influenza**

There are a billion new cases each year with up to a million deaths in the world. We fear a reprise of the Spanish flu but so far it hasn't happened. Influenza comes around every year, and every five or six years a more virulent strain appears. The flu epidemic of 2018 led to the deaths of forty thousand in the US, the highest ever recorded. The vaccine has variable efficacy that alters on a yearly basis.

10. **AIDS**

The most troublesome statistic about AIDS is that, of the thirty-eight million people estimated to be infected worldwide in 2019, 30 percent are unaware that they have the disease. It is at its worst in South and East Africa, which saw 44 percent of the new cases. Highly active antiretroviral therapy (HAART) effectively suppresses the infection, allowing the patient to live normally, but it must be taken for life. A cure or vaccine is still awaited.

11. **Mosquito-borne "rain forest viruses": dengue, chikungunya, Zika, and West Nile**

All of these infections are on the increase worldwide, particularly since 2010, mostly because of poor mosquito control leading to increasing numbers in a widening habitat plus increased travel.

12. **COVID-19**

The epidemic continues as of early 2021. Over 2.3 million have died to date.

GLOSSARY

Archaea: Single-celled organisms distinct from bacteria and eukaryotes that make up the third domain of life.

Autochtonous: Of a place, indigenous, rather than descended from migrants or colonists.

Cachexia: Weakness and wasting of the body from disease.

Chloroplast: Organelles in plants and algae that conduct photosynthesis.

Chorea: A neurological disorder characterized by jerky involuntary movements affecting the shoulders, legs, and face.

Cytokine: Small messenger proteins essential for immunity.

Dioecious: Having the male and female reproductive organs in separate individuals.

Endogenous: Growing or originating within an organism.

Epizootic: An epidemic, or outbreak of disease, in animals.

Genome: An entire set of genes of an individual (arranged in humans on chromosomes). There are twenty-three pairs of chromosomes in the nucleus of each cell (except for germ cells; see *meiosis*).

Gram stain: A method of staining bacteria named after Hans Christian Gram, a Dane who first performed his stain in 1884. It classifies bacteria into two large groups, Gram positive and Gram negative.

Meiosis: A type of cell division that leads to daughter cells with half the number of chromosomes of the parent cell.

Microbiome: The genetic material of all the microbes that live on and inside the human body.

Mitosis: A type of cell division in which the daughter cells have the same number and kind of chromosomes as the parent.

Pathogen: A bacterium, virus, or other microorganism that can cause a disease.

Sylvatic: Infections in wild animals, as opposed to domestic.

Zoonosis: A disease that can be transmitted to humans from animals.

FOR FURTHER READING

There is an extensive literature. I stopped counting at a hundred books and have listed twenty-one of my favorites. I have mixed history with science, fiction, and science fiction.

The History of the Peloponnesian War | Thucydides

Journal of the Plague Year | Daniel Defoe

The Decameron | Giovanni Boccaccio

Bleak House | Charles Dickens

Typhus | Anton Chekhov

An Enemy of the People | Henrik Ibsen

"The Masque of the Red Death" | Edgar Allan Poe

Rats, Lice and History | Hans Zinsser

Plagues and People | William H. McNeill

Love in the Time of Cholera | Gabriel García Márquez

The Siege of Krishnapur | J. G. Farrell

The American Plague | Molly Caldwell Crosby

Pox: Genius, Madness, and the Mysteries of Syphilis | Deborah Hayden

The Day of the Triffids | John Wyndham

And the Band Played On | Randy Shilts

Cutting For Stone | Abraham Verghese

Viruses: More Friends Than Foes | Karin Moelling

Shakespeare's Tremor and Orwell's Cough | John J. Ross

The Red Queen | Matt Ridley

The Fever | Sonia Shah

Who We Are and How We Got Here | David Reich

INDEX

ACKNOWLEDGMENTS

First, I must thank Bob Berman, aka Skyman Bob. I acknowledge unconditional gratitude. His enthusiasm, encouragement, and all-around support was such that this book would not have seen the light of day without him.

I thank Susan Brown for her unfailing friendship and advice.

To Duff McDonald I owe a huge debt. I have learned so much from one so young!

I would like to thank Dr. Richard Bird, Janet Pressley, Christopher Whatmore, and Rabbi Moshe Mones for valuable insights.

On the medical side, I wish to acknowledge the following physicians: the late Neville Southwell, FRCP, and the late James Willis, FRCP. They both showed me how to practice medicine without losing touch with the significance of disease and its human meaning.

By the same token, I want to thank David Warrell, Nicholas Woodhouse, Jens Otto Sieck, Ulla Sieck, and Zeev Weitz for friendship and insights.

I would like to thank my comrades-in-arms Catherine Allen, Anthony Guerrino, Charles Kutler, Bright Nkrumah, Marc Tack, and Andrew Yanofsky.

Thank you, Amy Bafumo, RN, for the long conversations we had about plagues.

Nurses are the unsung heroes of the medical profession. I acknowledge there would be no practice of medicine without them. If I were to single out a group to thank as examples of the whole, it would be the nurses who worked and still work in the Emergency Room and wards of the Kingston Hospital in New York State with professionalism and grace through the COVID-19 pandemic. I cannot name them all but will name those on the day shift in the ICU during the pandemic as representatives of the entire crew: Liz Beaulieu, Heather Cappa, Amber Carpino, Eric Christiansen, Stan Czaplak, Richelle DeGuzman, Danielle Deierlein, Kim Dyson, Nicole Hartigan, Linda Metcalf, Dianne Metsger, Mary Alice Mulstay, Erin Paul, Liz Senf, Jessica Simpson, and Courtney Vedder. Thank you.

Finally, I would like to thank my partner, Elaine Taylor, who has put up with my morbid preoccupations for the last five years with humor and love.

ABOUT THE AUTHOR

JOHN FROUDE was born in Sussex on the south coast of England and was educated at Steyning Grammar School and Guy's Hospital Medical School of the University of London. He worked in England, Nigeria, Uganda, Zimbabwe, Saudi Arabia, and Oman before finally settling in New York City during the AIDS epidemic. He worked at New York University for ten years.

He currently spends six months a year in Woodstock, New York, where he practices infectious disease medicine, and six months a year in Worthing, Sussex, where he writes.